Health Benefits of Vitamins

Types, Sources and Health Benefits of Vitamins

Written By: Dr. Alex Oselu Owiti;

B. Pharm, MT, M. Pharm, PhD

Copyright © 2021

All Rights Reserved

ISBN: 9781797685229

Statement

A part of the proceeds of this book will be designated to help feed the children of Africa, who are facing hunger due to issues in the food supply resulting from poverty, famine, and war.

Dedication

This book is dedicated to the children of Africa, who live with limited to no food due to abject poverty and violence, and to those who die in large numbers worldwide due to hunger and malnourishment.

Acknowledgment

Many people assisted me in the writing of this book. However, there are a few who are especially worth noting. Chief among them is my family. It is my concern for their health and longevity that makes me empathize with the fact that other people undoubtedly want their families to be healthy too. Indeed, the love and support showered upon me by my family gives me the inspiration to work in this field.

I also wish to acknowledge all of my colleagues, peers, and fellow academics in the field. I know that it is the combined result of all our efforts that produced the research for this book, in addition to the availability of in-depth information on exactly what Vitamins our body needs to operate at its optimal. I hope to keep working in this field alongside the rest of you so we can further the human condition together.

Lastly, I wish to acknowledge all those who have supported me over the years. Your encouragement helped develop confidence in my abilities to write this book. Your unwavering support means the world to me.

About the Author

Dr. Alex Oselu Owiti holds a PhD degree in Pharmaceutical Science (Pharmaceutics, Pharmacology and Toxicology) from the University of Missouri Kansas City-USA. He is an experienced pharmacist and researcher in the field of pharmacy and a board-certified medical technologist in USA. He also bears a bachelor's degrees in medical technology and Pharmacy and a master's degree in Pharmaceutical Science. In addition, he worked as professor at the schools of medicine in both California and Oklahoma, USA, as well as pharmacist in various pharmacies and hospitals. Currently, he is involved in development and research of various nano-formulations for delivery systems of different drugs, including anti-cancer medications.

Preface

The health benefits of Vitamins are numerous. But unfortunately, our lack of knowledge and limited awareness prevents us from benefiting from these vital super components present in our food. Many books of this kind are written in highly technical terms which makes it difficult for the general public to understand them. In this book, simple and more understandable words are used to elaborate and point out the types, sources and health benefits of Vitamins. This will enable readers at all levels of education worldwide to understand the concepts of this book.

This book is a guide which will enable the reader to grasp all the essential values of Vitamins, and hopefully, encourage the incorporation of them into the daily diet as needed.

Did you know that Vitamins can cure diseases?. This book explores the natural and organic world of Vitamins in the hopes of helping us all stay healthy.

Through this book, the author intends to help you, as

well as the children in Africa. A part of the proceeds of this book will be designated to feeding the children of Africa, who are endangered by malnourishment due to lack of food.

Contents

Dedication — *i*

Acknowledgment — *ii*

About The Author — *iv*

Preface — *v*

Chapter 1 . Vitamins — *1*

Chapter 2 . Vitamin A — *22*

Chapter 3 . Vitamins B1, B2, B3, B5 — *40*

Chapter 4 . Vitamin B6 — *62*

Chapter 5 . Vitamin B9 — *80*

Chapter 6 . Vitamin B12 — *101*

Chapter 7 . Vitamin C — *126*

Chapter 8 . Vitamin D — *155*

Chapter 9 . Vitamin E — *171*

Chapter 10 . Vitamin K — *185*

Page Left Blank Intentionally

Chapter 1

Vitamins

A Vitamin is an organic compound that is crucial to human beings and all the other living organisms. We all need these Vitamins in our bodies. They have a very important role to play inside us, as they have many advantages that have significant effects on our health.

Vitamins can be categorized in two ways: fat-soluble and water-soluble Vitamins. Vitamins A, D, E, and K belong to the fat-soluble category. They are stored in the fat tissues and the liver. They can stay in the body for as long as six months. When they are needed by a particular part of our body, they are transported to that part via blood and special carriers.

Vitamin B and C belong to the water-soluble category. They are not stored in the body. They travel in the bloodstream and need to be refilled on a frequent basis.

ALEX OSELU OWITI; B. PHARM, MT, M. PHARM, PHD

Vitamin A

Vitamin A has proven to be a very powerful antioxidant. It is highly effective in maintaining a clear vision. Apart from that, it plays a key role in neurological functions. It also helps to keep the skin healthy besides many other benefits. Vitamin A, like all other antioxidants, helps with fighting and reducing free radicals in the body; thus, reducing the damages to the body's systems.

Having food items in your diet that are rich in antioxidants helps reduce the aging process of the body. The antioxidant activity of Vitamin A also helps build and keep strong bones. Apart from keeping the bones healthy, antioxidants are also good for balancing the gene regulation and facilitating cell differentiation, preventing mutations and cancer development.

They also support immune functions. It is important to eat foods that are good sources of Vitamin A. Some sources of Vitamin A include milk, eggs, liver, carrots, and vegetables that are yellow or orange in color. Green, leafy vegetables are an especially good source.

Apart from the vision, skin, and bones, Vitamin A is also important for safeguarding the mucous membranes of several systems in our body, including digestive, respiratory, and urinary systems against infections. People who have complaints of long-term malabsorption usually have a deficiency of Vitamin A.

Deficiency of Vitamin A in our bodies can lead to poor eye health, premature skin damage, respiratory infections, and major complications during pregnancy.

Vitamin B (B1, B2, B3, B5)

Vitamin B is found in many foods. It belongs to the water-soluble category and is delicate and unstable in nature. It can be easily degraded, especially by alcohol and excess heat during the cooking process. Vitamin B is reduced when foods are processed. Some examples of processes that may lead to its degradation include milling, bread baking, and rice processing, which might end up eliminating most of the Vitamin nutrients.

Our body has limited room to store Vitamins B, except for Vitamin B9 and B12, which are kept in the liver. A person who has been on a terrible diet for more than a few months can develop a deficiency of Vitamin B. Therefore, it is important to include foods that are rich in Vitamin B as part of a healthy and balanced diet.

Vitamin B1

Vitamin B1 is also known as thiamin. Its basic function is to help during the conversion of glucose into energy, besides being helpful with nerve functioning. Some of the good sources of thiamin are whole meal grains and legumes. It is also found in seeds, such as sesame, wheatgerm, nuts, and yeast. In some countries like Australia, it is obligatory to have white and whole meal flour that is fortified with thiamin.

It is naturally found in some foods, while it is added to other food products. It is also easily available as a dietary supplement. It plays a vital role in energy production metabolism and is helpful with development, growth, and the proper functioning of body tissues and cells.

The deficiency of thiamin is very common in countries that have a high consumption rate of white rice. Western countries consume large amounts of alcohol and, usually, have a rather unhealthy diet. They are also likely to suffer the Vitamin B1 deficiency. Thiamin deficiency symptoms are very noticeable. Some of these are irritability, confusion, an imbalance in arm and leg coordination, weakening of muscles, fatigue, and lethargy. The small intestine absorbs Thiamin that is ingested from food and dietary supplements. This happens through active transport at different nutritional doses. It also happens by unassertive diffusion at pharmacologic doses.

Wet and dry beriberi are two diseases caused by the deficiency of Vitamin B1. Wet beriberi can lead to heart failure, whereas dry beriberi can lead to decreased muscle strength. It can also result in muscle paralysis if adequate attention is not paid.

Vitamin B2

Vitamin B2 is also known as riboflavin. It is essentially responsible for producing energy in the body. It also helps maintain healthy vision and healthy skin. Some of the best sources of riboflavin are milk, yogurt, cottage cheese, wholegrain bread, cereals, egg – especially egg whites, leafy green vegetables, meat, yeast, liver, and kidney.

Deficiency of riboflavin is very rare and is usually placed alongside deficiencies of other B group Vitamins. People who are most likely to develop a deficiency of riboflavin are those who consume large amounts of alcohol and other alcohol-based beverages. It can also happen to people who do not have milk or milk products as a part of their diets. The symptoms of riboflavin deficiency include inflammation of the tongue. In this situation, the tongue becomes painful, smooth and turns purple-red in color. Cracks and intense redness can also occur on the tongue, as well as on the corners and around the mouth. Other symptoms include anxiety, inflamed eyelids, and sensitivity to light, apart from reddening of the cornea and rashes on the skin.

Some people take riboflavin orally to maintain healthy hair, skin, and nails. They also do so to slow aging, for canker sores, multiple sclerosis, and memory loss – including Alzheimer's disease, high blood pressure, burns, liver diseases, and sickle cell anemia.

Vitamin B3

Vitamin B3 is also known as niacin. It is essential for the process of turning carbohydrates, fat, and alcohol into energy, which can then be used by the body. It helps with keeping the skin healthy. It also supports major systems of the body, including nervous and digestive systems. Niacin is very stable when it is exposed to heat, so a very small portion of it loses its nutritional value during cooking.

Foods that are rich sources of niacin include meat, fish, poultry, milk, eggs, cereals, nuts, mushrooms, wholegrain bread, and foods that contain a higher quantity of protein.

When consumed in large quantities, niacin has a drug-like effect on the blood fats and the nervous system. Its side effects include flushes, itching, nausea, and the possibility of severe liver damage; even though positive changes may be witnessed in the blood fats.

Niacin deficiency is called pellagra. It is common among people who consume abnormally large amounts of alcohol. It is also common in people whose diets consist exclusively of corn. Some other causes of pellagra are interlinked with problems of digestion, where the body becomes unable to absorb niacin effectively. The primary symptoms of pellagra are known as the three Ds. These Ds are dementia, diarrhea, and dermatitis. Other noticeable symptoms of pellagra are inflammation and swelling of the tongue, irritability, loss of appetite, mental confusion, weakness, and dizziness. If not treated in due time, pellagra can lead to death.

Vitamin B5

Vitamin B5 is also known as pantothenic acid. It is important in mobilizing the carbohydrates, protein, fats, and alcohol, as well as facilitating their metabolism. It is also beneficial during the production of red blood cells in the body, as well as the steroid hormones.

Foods that contain high quantities of pantothenic acid include liver, meat, milk, kidneys, eggs, yeast, peanuts, and legumes. The deficiency of pantothenic acid is extremely rare and uncommon. The symptoms that point to the deficiency of pantothenic acid include a loss of appetite, lack of proper sleep, constipation, fatigue, vomiting, and distress in the intestine.

Pantothenic acid is taken orally as a medicine for diseases like osteoarthritis, rheumatoid arthritis, Parkinson's disease, nerve pain, premenstrual syndrome (PMS), and enlarged prostate, among others. It is also used for the treatment of physical and mental stress and anxiety. It is used for reducing signs of aging, lowering vulnerability to infections – such as colds and others, retarded growth, and shingles. It is also effective for skin disorders, and is used for stimulating the adrenal glands, chronic fatigue syndrome, salicylate toxicity, streptomycin neurotoxicity, dizziness, and wound healing.

Pantothenic acid can also be applied externally; for example, in dexpanthenol, a creamy formulation that is made from Vitamin B5. It can be used for the treatment of itching on the skin and healing mild eczemas, among other skin conditions besides insect bites and stings, poison ivy, rashes from diapers, and general skin acne. It can also be effective for treating skin reactions to radiation therapy.

ALEX OSELU OWITI; B. PHARM, MT, M. PHARM, PHD

Vitamin B6

Vitamin B6 is also known as pyridoxine. It is important for metabolizing proteins and carbohydrates. It is critical in forming red blood cells and certain brain chemicals. It has an impact on the processes of the brain and its development, the immune function, and steroid hormone activity.

Foods that are rich in pyridoxine include legumes, cereal grains, green leafy vegetables, normal fish and shellfish, meat and poultry, nuts, liver, and fruits. Consuming excessive quantities of pyridoxine, especially in the form of supplements, can result in harmful levels accumulating in the body and severely damaging the nerves.

The symptoms of unadvised excessive intake of pyridoxine include difficulty with walking and numbness in the hands and feet. It can lead to severe nerve damage when large doses of Vitamin B6 are consumed over a considerable period of time.

Pyridoxine deficiency is common among people who drink a lot of alcohol regularly. It is more common in women who take contraceptive pills and older people who have thyroid diseases. Noticeable symptoms of the deficiency include lack of proper sleep, anemia, the smoothening of the tongue, the cracking of mouth corners, irritability, twitching of the muscles, dermatitis, convulsions, and confusion.

It has been discovered that Vitamin B6 can prove to be highly beneficial in curing and treating carpal tunnel syndrome and PMS. It is advised to consult your doctor or a medical professional before taking it.

Vitamin B9

Vitamin B9 is also known as folate or folic acid. Folate is important because it is required for the formation of red blood cells. Red blood cells carry oxygen around the body. They assist in the development of the fetal nervous system, as well as the healthy DNA synthesis and growth of cells. Expectant women should have a diet that is rich in folic acid for proper development of their fetuses.

Some of the foods that are good sources of folate are leafy green vegetables, legumes, seeds, liver, poultry, eggs, cereal, and citrus fruits. Since 2009, all flour used in bread has been fortified with folic acid, including the flour that is sold as organic.

Folate is usually thought to be non-toxic, even though it has been discovered that taking an excess of 1000 mg/day of folate over a period of time can lead to malaise, irritability, and intestinal dysfunction. The primary risk that excessive consumption of folate can pose is that it may make it difficult to diagnose deficiency of other vitamins particularly Vitamin B12 deficiency. It is recommended to consume these Vitamins in moderate quantities.

The symptoms of folate deficiency include extreme fluctuations in weight, tiredness, weakness, and fatigue. Anemia related to folate deficiency is called megaloblastic anemia, and it is another major symptom. An elevated risk of neural tube defects, such as spina bifida for babies during pregnancy, is also a symptom of folate deficiency. This is why pregnant women should include foods in their diets that contain Vitamin B9 (folic acid). It has an important role during development and maturation process of red blood cells. If consumed wisely in the right amount and at the right time, it can help the baby develop a proper circulatory system while still in the womb.

Vitamin B12

Vitamin B12 is also known as cyanocobalamin. It is beneficial in producing and maintaining the myelin sheath that surrounds the nerve cells. It also helps with retaining mental abilities, formation of red blood cells, and, during the process of breaking down fatty and amino acids, producing energy. Vitamin B12 works closely with Vitamin B9 (folate) because both are interdependent on each other to work properly and carry out their respective functions.

Some foods that are rich in B12 Vitamins are liver, meat, milk, cheese, eggs, and every other food item that comes directly from animals.

The elderly people are more susceptible to Vitamin B12 deficiency. Vitamin B12 deficiency is also common among vegans and vegetarians because the main source of Vitamin B12, as mentioned above, is animals. This means that this deficiency may be passed on to babies who are breastfed by vegan mothers.

There are many symptoms of Vitamin B12 deficiencies, which include tiredness, fatigue, and loss of appetite, which may lead to weight loss, heart palpitations, shortness of breath, vision loss, and the smoothening of the tongue. There are also mental symptoms such as depression and memory loss.

You are more likely to develop a B12 deficiency if you have a condition called 'atrophic gastritis,' in which the lining of the stomach wall gets thinner, and if you are suffering from pernicious anemia. This makes it difficult for the body to absorb Vitamin B12. You can also have a B12 deficiency if you have medical conditions like Crohn's and celiac diseases, bacterial growth, parasites that have a direct effect on your small intestine. Also, from Graves' disease, or lupus, all of which are immune system disorders.

Vitamin C

Vitamin C is also known as ascorbic acid. It belongs to the water-soluble category of Vitamins. It comes with antioxidant properties that neutralizes free radicals and lowers the risk of inflammation and other diseases. It is also needed by our bodies to synthesize important compounds. An example of these compounds is collagen, which is a type of structural protein that makes up connective tissue and also helps with healing wounds and bruises. Vitamin C is also important because it produces other compounds, such as L-carnitine and neurotransmitters.

Continuous research has discovered a large number of possible Vitamin C advantages. It has been found that adding Vitamin C to our diets can give better results to our skin. Other than that, it can help boost immunity and protect the body against certain medical conditions. It also helps with the prevention of anemia, improves the overall condition of the heart, and lowers the chances of getting gout, among many other benefits.

Vitamin C is present in almost all fruits and vegetables. Some of these fruits are kiwis, oranges, strawberries, papaya, pineapple, grapefruit, and mangoes, among others. Vegetables are a good source of Vitamin C, which includes green leaves, bell peppers, broccoli, Brussel sprouts, tomatoes, spinach, and many others.

Vitamin C deficiency in the body can result in a medical condition called scurvy. There are multiple symptoms of scurvy. Some of the symptoms are slow healing of wounds, getting bruised too easily, bleeding and swelling of gums, fatigue, frequent nosebleeds, and dry scaly skin, to name a few.

Vitamin D

Vitamin D belongs to the fat-soluble category. It is stored in the liver and fatty tissues of our bodies, which means that body fat can absorb and store Vitamin D.

It has different characteristics from other Vitamins because our body makes enough of it on its own without depending on food items.

Our bodies mobilize the stored Vitamin D when we are exposed to sunlight, which converts it into chemicals ready for use in the body. The cholesterol that is present in our skin converts pre-Vitamin D and turns it into usable Vitamin D3, which is also called Vitamin D. The Vitamin D travels through the kidneys and liver into our bloodstream. It is then converted into calcitriol, which is a biologically active and ready-to-be-used substance.

Vitamin D turns into a hormone inside the body called the secosteroid hormone. Since Vitamin D is antecedent to a steroid hormone, it has an impact on the structure of our skeleton, as well as our blood pressure, immune system, mood, the functioning of the brain, and our body's ability to guard itself against cancer.

While the basic source of Vitamin D is the sunlight, there are substitutes for it. These great sources include: eggs, raw milk and fishes, such as halibut, mackerel, carp fish, eel, salmon, whitefish, rainbow trout, swordfish, sardines, tuna, and oil from the liver of cod. Apart from fishes, there are other sources like maitake and portobello mushrooms, both of which are exposed directly to UV light from the sun.

Symptoms that point to the deficiency of Vitamin D are weakness, chronic fatigue, bouts of depression, trouble sleeping, anxiety, and weakening of bones, which can lead to bone breakage, weak immune system, inflammation, and swelling.

Vitamin E

ALEX OSELU OWITI; B. PHARM, MT, M. PHARM, PHD

Vitamin E belongs to the fat-soluble category. Like many other Vitamins, it also has antioxidant properties that prevent comprehensive damage to particular fats in the body. They are important for health and also help with slowing down the aging process. Vitamin E is important for the proper functioning of several organs, along with enzymatic activities and neurological processes.

There are many benefits of Vitamin E. It helps balance our cholesterol levels, fights free radicals, helps our body by preventing diseases, repairs damaged skin, thickens hair, balances hormones, helps reduce premenstrual syndromes (PMS) symptoms, improves eyesight, combats Alzheimer's, improves effects of medical procedures on the body – making them more effective – improves physical endurance, and strengthens muscles, among other improvements. It is also critical during pregnancy for the growth and development of the baby. It has been discovered that Vitamin E has properties that can cure cancer.

Structurally, Vitamin E is made up of four tocopherols and four tocotrienols. Thus, it is especially important for expectant women, fetuses, toddlers, infants, and older people. The recommended amount of Vitamin E for daily consumption by adults is 15 milligrams per day, according to the USDA.

Some of the best sources of Vitamin E are sunflower seeds, almonds, hazelnuts, wheat germ, mangoes, avocados, butternut squash, broccoli, spinach, kiwi, and tomatoes.

There are a number of symptoms that can point to a deficiency of Vitamin E. Some of these are the weakening of muscles, loss of muscle mass, abnormal movements of the eye, problems in vision and eyesight, and unsteady walking.

Vitamin K

Vitamin K belongs to the fat-soluble category. It plays an important role in blood clotting, metabolism of the bones, and regulating levels of calcium in the blood. Our body requires Vitamin K to make a protein and clotting factor called prothrombin. It helps with the clotting of blood and our bone metabolism. People who utilize medications such as warfarin or Coumadin for blood thinning purposes should never begin taking Vitamin K without consulting their doctor or physician.

Vitamin K deficiency is uncommon, but a lack of Vitamin K can increase clotting time, resulting in severe hemorrhaging, and even uncontrolled bleeding in some cases. Vitamin K has a number of benefits. These include the improvement of bone health, cognitive health, and keeping the heart healthy.

There are a number of foods that are rich in Vitamin K. Some of these are leafy green vegetables, such as kale and Swiss chard, as well as vegetable oils and fruits. Others include parsley, natto, collard greens, spinach, soybean oil, grapes, and hard-boiled eggs. Another type of Vitamin K called K2, or menaquinones, can be found in meat, dairy products, and eggs.

In general, there are many symptoms that point to the deficiency of Vitamin K. These are easy bruising, blood oozing from nose or gums, uncontrolled bleeding from wounds, injuries, injection, and surgical sites, heavy menstrual periods, bleeding from the gastrointestinal tract, and bleeding in urine or stool.

After understanding the basics of each type of Vitamin

highlighted in this chapter, we will discuss, in the following chapters, multiple food sources, and the significance of each for the human body, in greater detail.

ALEX OSELU OWITI; B. PHARM, MT, M. PHARM, PHD

Chapter 2

Vitamin A

Vitamin A is one of the most important nutrients for the human body. The term "Vitamin A" is a collective terminology for retinoid. Retinoid is a biologically mobile compound. It is found in both animal and plant tissues naturally. Vitamin A acts as a crucial fat-soluble Vitamin and a powerful antioxidant. It is imperative to get sufficient amounts of Vitamin A in your body to maintain a proper and healthy state of your body. Vitamin A is highly effective in having a healthy skin that is fresh and clear.

It is also an important nutrient for preventing your body from diseases, by keeping strong immunity and healthy bones. It has an important role in maintaining clear and steady vision, the neurological function of our body, as well as many other benefits. It is an important factor in the process of decreasing inflammation in our body through combating free radical damage, like every other antioxidant does.

Vitamin A exists in two primary types. The first is active Vitamin A, which is also called Retinol. Retinyl esters are a result of Retinol. The second type of Vitamin A is Beta-carotene. Retinol is found in foods that come from animals. It is a kind of a "pre-formed" Vitamin A that is ready to be used by the body directly. The beta-carotene Vitamin A is in the form of pro-Vitamin A called carotenoids. It is found in fruits and vegetables of various colors. Beta-carotene and other kinds of carotenoids that are found in plants and plants-based products first need to be changed to retinol so that it is ready to be used by the body. Palmitate is another type of Vitamin A. It comes in capsule form.

Benefits of Vitamin A

Improves Eye Health

The capability to enhance our vision and keep our eyes healthy is one of the most commonly known and famous benefits of Vitamin A. This is because it is an important part of the rhodopsin molecule. The rhodopsin molecule is activated when our retina is exposed to light. This delivers a signal to the brain, and that is how we are able to see. Beta-carotene is responsible for the prevention of macular degeneration, which is one of the most common and leading reasons of blindness related to old age. People who had the daily intake of multivitamins that were high in Vitamin A, Vitamin C, Vitamin E, zinc, copper – and simultaneously had a higher possibility of attracting the disease – had a 25 percent lesser risk of macular degeneration at an advanced level during a yearly period, according to a study printed in the Archives of Ophthalmology.

Improves Immunity

Vitamin A has an important role in immune health. It has been noted that Vitamin A can be effective in preventing illnesses and infections. Vitamin A deficiency can result in weak immunity and even changes the function of immune cells. Vitamin A is helpful in stopping the regeneration of the mucosal barriers, leading to a reduced susceptibility to infections.

Relieves Inflammation

Beta-carotene is a powerful and a highly effective antioxidant in the body. It helps in decreasing the collection of toxic free radicals and stopping oxidative damage to cells, thus reducing inflammation. The anti-inflammatory effects of Vitamin A and beta-carotene can have long lasting results on our health because inflammation is the cause of a number of persistent conditions such as cancer, heart diseases and diabetes, to name a few examples. Other diseases include Alzheimer's and Parkinson's, which are neurodegenerative in nature, as well as Crohn's disease and rheumatoid arthritis.

Healthier Skin

Vitamin A is known for its skin nourishing abilities. Dermatologists often prescribe it to help in fighting acne and other blemishes. Applying retinol on the affected areas on the skin improves the lines of ageing and wrinkles. It also improves the skin's ability to heal from injuries.

Vitamin A can also be helpful in the cure of a wide range of skin related issues because of its anti-inflammatory properties. Studies have revealed that retinoid can be therapeutic for day-to-day skin issues, like psoriasis, eczema and acne.

Combating Cancer

It is said that there is a strong link between what you eat and how it can or cannot cause cancer. Increasing your intake of foods that are rich in Vitamin A can help in the prevention of cancer cells' development in your body. Retinoid has displayed properties of blocking abnormal growth of skin, bladder, breast, prostate and lung cancer cells in *in vitro* studies. Large intakes of retinoic acid can be harmful to cells, so it is advised to consume Vitamin A moderately through food and food sources in our daily diet over a period of time. Consumption in moderation is always a good idea to see better and prompt results.

Healthier Bones

Vitamin A is a crucial nutrient for the healthy and

positive growth of bones. The adequate consumption of Vitamin A is important because in both cases – of excessive levels of consumption than what is advised or lower than what is advised – can have a negative effect on the overall health of the bones. Blood retinol levels were visibly lesser in older women that were suffering from osteoporosis when a comparison was made in a control group. The final results also displayed that lower retinol levels were related to a decreased density of bone minerals in the femur bone.

Reduces Cholesterol

Cholesterol is a lipoprotein substance that is found throughout our bodies. Our bodies require cholesterol to work and operate normally because it is involved in hormone synthesis. It is the base of the foundation of our cell membranes. There are two types of cholesterol, namely High-density lipoprotein HDL – also known as good cholesterol, and Low-density Lipoprotein LDL – also called bad Cholesterol. An excess amount of bad cholesterol can take up space in our blood vessels, resulting in the vessels becoming narrow and hard, which elevates the risk of heart disease. Studies reveal that consuming sufficient amounts of Vitamin A in our daily diets can help in lowering cholesterol in our bodies naturally, which would improve our heart health.

Spurs Growth and Development

Vitamin A is important for ideal growth and development during all the important phases of our lives. It is known to be one of the best Vitamins for women and their health. A deficiency of Vitamin A is associated with depressed immune functions, higher rates of mortality and even larger risks of mother-to-child transfers of HIV-1 among infected expectant women. The American Pediatrics Association states that Vitamin A as one of the most crucial micronutrients during pregnancy. It is extremely important for lung functioning and baby maturation. Beta-carotene is also effective in stopping developmental disorders for fetuses and breast-feeding babies.

Repairs Tissue

Adding foods in your diet that are rich in Vitamin A is imperative for repairing damaged tissues and the regeneration of cells. It is important to consume enough Vitamin A for these purposes. It has also been said that Vitamin A can assist in healing wounds. Research reveals that prior treatment using retinoid helped in improving the wound healing process after undergoing facial surgeries or procedures, depending on the severity of the case.

Prevents Kidney Stones

Kidney stones can be an extremely painful condition. They form in our kidneys and then rapidly grow in size in the bladder. They can lead to medical symptoms, including constant urination, pain in the abdomen area, severe discomfort and hematuria, which causes blood to appear in the urine. Kidney stones can cause serious infections and difficulties when left untreated. Some cases are so bad that they require immediate medical attention. According to some studies, Vitamin A can help in stopping kidney stones from forming. One of those studies looked closely at the connection between levels of Vitamin A in the human body and kidney stones forming in children. They concluded that higher traces of calcium oxalate in the urine lead to a higher risk of formation of kidney stones.

Symptoms of Vitamin A Deficiency

As discussed earlier, Vitamin A plays a role in maintaining healthy vision, skin as well as bone growth. It is also important for the protection of mucous membranes of bodily systems, such as respiratory and digestive systems. It is also effective in the prevention of infections in the urinary tracts.

People who suffer from long-term malabsorption of fats are more likely to develop a deficiency of Vitamin A. Individuals with leaky gut syndrome, celiac diseases, inflammatory bowel disease, pancreatic and immune disorders, or addiction to alcohol are also at a threat of developing Vitamin A deficiency.

Vitamin A deficiency is most common in developing

countries. Indeed, it is very uncommon in the United States. One of the initial signs of Vitamin A deficiency is blindness during the night. If left untreated, it can lead to permanent damage to the eyesight. Vitamin A deficiency also invites diseases that cause infections such as measles and pneumonia, which can prove to be very dangerous.

Compulsive drinkers are likely to develop Vitamin A deficiencies. They should make it a point to include foods in their diets that are rich sources of Vitamin A. They should also try to reduce their consumption of alcohol to avoid any serious complications. Some doctors also prescribe supplements in such situations, but those may not be a smart decision for alcoholics. That is because our liver is the storage area of Vitamin A. Any current damage to the liver can make them susceptible to the toxicity and harmfulness of Vitamin A. The immediate attention and care of a doctor is crucial.

There are a number of other symptoms as well that point towards Vitamin A deficiency. These are as follows:

- Dry lips
- Thick or scaly skin
- Damaged immune system

- Slow growth in children
- Night blindness
- Bitot's spots, which is the condition of building up of Keratin on the conjunctiva
- Xerophthalmia, which is a condition in which the conjunctiva and the cornea dries up

Sources of Vitamin A

The richest animal source of retinols is beef liver. Three ounces of liver provides over 27000 IU (International Units). That is far more than what one needs during an entire day. The toxicity will not prove to be a problem until such high consumption happens on a daily basis. In addition to beef liver, high amounts of Vitamin A can also be found in dairy products (eggs, cheese, yogurt, and milk) and fish (salmon, mackerel and Bluefin tuna).

The best natural sources of carotenoids are, and always will be, fruits and vegetables. Carotenoid content is often found in abundance in red, orange, yellow and dark green fruits and vegetables. These include, but are not limited to, carrots, spinach, kale, butternut squash, cantaloupe, mangos, sweet potatoes and pumpkins.

Ever wondered why carrots are recommended for people with depleting eyesight? It is because these Vitamin A-rich food sources provide you with beta-carotene (a kind of Vitamin A) that promotes better vision and overall improved eye health. Studies have also revealed that Vitamin A consumption prevents renal scarring (damaged kidneys) in people. And that's just a couple of benefits of Vitamin A consumption.

Increasing the intake of foods and food sources that are rich in Vitamin A is the ideal way to obtain the benefits and goodness of this vital nutrient. Below are the best foods that are bursting with the goodness of Vitamin A. Incorporating these in your daily meals will ensure that you have consumed and are satisfying your required intake of Vitamin A on a daily basis.

- Butternut squash
- Sweet potato
- Kale
- Carrots
- Beef Liver

- Spinach
- Dried apricots
- Broccoli
- Butter
- Egg yolks

There are some other foods as well that have abundant Vitamin A. They include: Green peas, red bell peppers, tomatoes, full fat raw milk, cod liver oil, mangoes, cantaloupe, papaya and oatmeal. Additionally, herbs that are rich in Vitamin A like basil and paprika are some of these foods.

Increasing Vitamin A in Our Diet

5000 IU is the advised Vitamin A dosage per day for adults and children that are over the age of four. An IU of retinol equals roughly 0.3 µg of Retinol Activity Equivalents (RAE). In the same way, one IU of beta-carotene is about 0.15 µg of RAE when consumed through supplements.

It can be very simple, convenient, and even appetizing to meet your daily required intake of Vitamin A by just increasing your daily consumption of fresh fruits and vegetables, and adding a serving or two of them in your daily meals depending on the requirement and needs of Vitamin A. A simple way to do that is to roast a handful of carrots as a delicious side for your meal. You may have meat as the entrée, or you could make a kale salad to go with your main course.

Another way is to slice open a butternut squash and bake it in the oven for a couple of minutes by adding butter from grass-fed or herb-fed animals. These are just some of the ways in which you can increase your intake of Vitamin A. You can come up with your own recipes and ideas to get enough Vitamin A, while keeping things interesting during your meal times. Remember, a variety of colored fruits and vegetables will always be beneficial for you.

They will ensure you are provided with your much-needed quantity of Vitamin A, leaving you feeling fresh, energized and ready to take on the day. Adding fruits in your breakfast and in your snacks is a great way to get the best possible benefits of Vitamin A.

There are a number of tablets and supplements on the market that can be consumed to get your required intake of Vitamin A. Many people prefer doing it that way, substituting supplements for food, because they are of the opinion that it is a much quicker way of getting the required intake of Vitamin A. This will continue to remain the secondary way of doing so. The best way of increasing your consumption of Vitamin A will always be through eating your fruits and vegetables.

These are the food sources that are rich enough to give you the benefits of Vitamin A naturally. They have a higher quotient of Vitamin A in them and can be counted on to give you the maximum benefits. Studies and research have revealed that supplementing Vitamins through 'alternative' methods, such as beta-carotene for Vitamin A, are linked to an increased risk of cancer in a massive chunk of the population.

Precautions While Taking Vitamin A

Vitamin A has a number of benefits and is good for our

health. But like all things, it also has its fair share of disadvantages. One must know the right balance between consuming enough of it and too much of it. As is the rule for everything else, moderation is key here.

Vitamin A, when consumed in high quantities, can result in doing more harm than good to our bodies. Vitamin A has been linked to defects and complications in birth, decreased bone density, and liver problems when consumed in higher quantities through supplementation or when combined with other antioxidants. The harmful quotient of Vitamin A can also lead to symptoms such as jaundice, nausea, hair loss, irritability, vomiting, food poisoning and appetite loss.

Make it a point to get an opinion from your doctor or consult them first when you decide to use Vitamin A supplements. It is advised that one should have low dosage intake and it is better if you rely on food-based sources as supplements as much as possible. People who are heavy drinkers, are chain smokers, are suffering from liver and kidney failures and other diseases are strongly advised to not consume Vitamin A supplements at all unless they have had a proper checkup and their doctor, or a certified medical professional, has advised them to take them.

Taking a supplement without consulting with your doctor can be a major medical mistake which may cause self-harm. It should be noted that Vitamin A can also react with certain medications and drugs, including some blood thinners, contraceptive or birth control pills, and certain cancer treatments.

It should be remembered that Vitamin A comes under the category of fat-soluble Vitamins, and therefore should always be taken with fat to ensure maximum absorption. A certain dietary intake of protein is necessary for producing these binding proteins, so deficient protein intake may lead to damaged Vitamin A function and a lack of absorption. One should go for food sources and combine them with a well-balanced diet that is rich in foods that have a higher quantity of nutrients to stop issues with over-dosage of Vitamin A or hypervitaminosis. This also helps in maximizing your health and making sure that the level of Vitamin A in your body stays at a required level.

Chapter 3

Vitamins B1, B2, B3, B5

The Vitamins in the B group are present in many foods that we consume on a regular basis. They belong to the water-soluble category and are delicate in nature. They can easily be destroyed, especially by alcohol and during cooking. Vitamin B is also reduced when foods are processed. Bread, rice, and flour are some examples that lose most nutrients as opposed to the whole grain options.

Our body has a very limited room to store the B group Vitamins, except for B12 and folate, which stay in the liver once ingested. A person that has been on an unhealthy diet for a couple of months can develop a deficiency of Vitamins from the B group. Hence, it is important to include foods that are rich in Vitamin B as part of a healthy and balanced diet.

ALEX OSELU OWITI; B. PHARM, MT, M. PHARM, PHD

Vitamin B1

Vitamin B1 is a co-enzyme utilized by our bodies to mobilize the food we eat through metabolism, which provides our body with the energy to live and perform day-to-day tasks. This is also important for maintaining a healthy condition of our hearts and nerve functions. Vitamin B1 is also known as thiamine. It is essential for digesting foods and extracting the required energy from the diet by turning the nutrients into usable energy in the form of 'ATP'.

Studies have shown that thiamine plays a structural role in the proper functioning of the nervous system. Vitamin B1 is the source of essential building blocks to nerve cells. These building blocks are required for the production of energy and increased blood flow to the neural tissues.

Thiamine is utilized when it is combined with other B-category Vitamins that form Vitamin B Complex. It regulates important functions and tasks of the cardiovascular system, along with the endocrine system and the digestive system. It comes under the category of water-soluble Vitamins and is used in almost every single one of the cells that are present in our body. It is also vital in sustaining high levels of energy, along with a healthy metabolism.

Thiamine deficiency can lead to problems in our health and body, such as weakness, chronic fatigue, heart complications, nerve damage, and psychosis. Thiamine is present in many foods that are consumed on a daily basis. These include yeasts, a number of whole grains, beans, nuts, and meat. Thiamine is also present in many Vitamin B supplement products of their complex nature.

According to the USDA, the required intake of thiamine for adults is 1.2 mg/day for men and 1.1 mg/day for women. It is said that a majority of adults complete this requirement. Some adults even consume double or triple the intake of thiamine when consumed in the form of supplements. Thiamine deficiency occurs very rarely in developed nations, but continues to prevail in underdeveloped countries.

Symptoms of Vitamin B1 Deficiency

The signs of a thiamine deficiency from a medical perspective include:

- Colitis
- Ongoing digestive problems, such as diarrhea
- Nerve damage
- Mental changes, such as apathy or depression
- Cardiovascular effects, such as an enlarged heart
- Nerve inflammation (neuritis)
- Fatigue and tiredness
- Decrease in short-term memory
- Confusion
- Irritability
- Muscle weakness
- Anorexia or rapid weight loss
- Poor appetite

Thiamine deficiency can lead to a condition called beriberi. It has been recorded in populations for over a thousand years, or perhaps longer. Beriberi is a medical condition characterized by muscle wasting and intense cardiovascular problems, like an enlarged heart. Countries such as the United States have witnessed thiamine deficiency mostly in alcoholics as of late. This is called Wernicke-Korsakoff syndrome. Alcoholics that suffer from the condition also complain about not feeling hungry or not eating enough food. This is one of the primary reasons that lead to thiamine deficiency in the first place.

Sources of Vitamin B1

The most powerful and rich food sources of thiamine include different kinds of beans, nuts, seeds, and spirulina powder made from seaweed. Then, there is yeast and nutritional yeast – a seasoning commonly used by vegetarians because the taste resembles cheese. Some types of meat organs, including liver, also contain smaller amounts of thiamine.

Thiamine is most commonly present in most whole grain, such as oats and barley, as well as grain-enriched products such as rice, pasta, bread, and cereal grain. These foods are enriched with thiamine, which is added to the food through synthetic processes.

While some of these foods do naturally contain thiamine

when consumed in their whole, unprocessed form, a lot of the Vitamin is lost during the refining process and therefore must be added back later. You will see words like 'enriched' or 'fortified' when it comes to products where thiamine is added to the food synthetically. Whole foods like nuts, beans, and seeds naturally contain a high amount of thiamine, unlike products that are highly processed.

There are some other food sources of thiamine.

- Nutritional yeast
- Seaweed
- Sunflower seeds
- Macadamia nuts
- Black beans
- Lentils
- Organic edamame
- Soybeans
- Navy beans
- White beans
- Green split peas

- Pinto beans
- Mung beans
- Beef liver
- Asparagus
- Brussel sprouts

Vitamin B2

Vitamin B2 is also known as Riboflavin. It is primarily responsible for producing energy in the body. It helps with maintaining healthy vision and healthy skin. Some of the best sources of riboflavin are milk, yogurt, cottage cheese, whole grain bread and cereals, eggs – especially egg whites, leafy green vegetables, meat, yeast, liver, and kidney.

Riboflavin deficiency is very rare. People who are most likely to develop a deficiency of riboflavin are those who consume large amounts of alcohol and other alcohol-based beverages. It can also happen to people who do not have milk or milk products as a part of their diets.

The symptoms of riboflavin deficiency include the

tongue getting inflamed. In this situation, the tongue becomes painful, smoothens, and turns a color of purple-red. Cracks and intense redness can also happen to the tongue, as well as corners and around the mouth. Other symptoms include anxiety, inflamed eyelids, and sensitivity to light, apart from reddening of the cornea and rashes on the skin.

Some people also take riboflavin orally to maintain healthy hair, skin, and nails, to slow aging, for canker sores, multiple sclerosis, and memory loss – including Alzheimer's disease, high blood pressure, burns, liver disease, and sickle cell anemia. Many people consume riboflavin orally because they want quick results.

A Vitamin B2 or riboflavin deficiency is uncommon in developed countries that continue to make breakthroughs in medicines and treatments for diseases. It is very rarely found in western countries because many refined carbohydrates are protected with riboflavin, according to a study carried out by USDA. Foods such as eggs and meat are a powerful source of Vitamin B2 and can be included in your daily diet for fast results.

The RDA for male adults is 1.3 mg in a day and 1.1 mg

for female adults. Children and toddlers need a lesser quantity of Vitamin B2. More Vitamin B2 might be necessary in order to help correct the underlying problems for individuals who are suffering from anemia, migraines, eye disorders, and thyroid dysfunction.

Symptoms of Vitamin B2 Deficiency

Some common symptoms associated with a lack of Vitamin B2 include:

- Inflamed mouth and tongue
- Sore throat
- Swelling of mucous membranes
- Changes in mood, such as increased anxiety and signs of depression
- Anemia
- Fatigue
- Nerve damage
- A sluggish metabolism
- Mouth or lip sores or cracks

- Skin inflammation
- Skin disorders, especially ones that happen on the nose and face

Sources of Vitamin B2

Some of the several sources of Vitamin B2 include:

- Almonds
- Beef or lamb meat (grass-fed)
- Tempeh, which is fermented soy
- Mackerel fish
- Liver (from lamb, beef, veal, turkey, or chicken)
- Eggs
- Seaweed
- Organ meat, including beef or lamb kidneys
- Mollusks/Cuttlefish
- Organic feta cheese
- Tahini/sesame seed paste

Riboflavin is usually found in the most fortified whole grains and enriched carbohydrate products, including bread, cereal, granola bar, and pasta. Normally, these foods are enriched with Vitamins and minerals, including riboflavin, after they are processed. Many of the naturally occurring nutrients are either removed or destroyed from these food sources.

The main reason most adults are able to meet their daily requirement for riboflavin in most situations, and avoid riboflavin deficiency, is that they most commonly consume packaged and refined carbohydrate products in their day-to-day diets.

Products that synthetically add Vitamins and minerals have the words 'enriched' or 'fortified' printed on their packaging. This is not the case with unprocessed products that naturally contain Vitamin B. These include meat, eggs, and sea vegetables.

There are multiple benefits of riboflavin. Some of the most important ones are:

- It is proven to help prevent headaches, including migraines. It is very effective in curing and soothing headaches.

- It helps maintain healthy eye vision.
- It helps prevent and treat anemia.
- It is important for maintaining proper energy levels.
- It is rich in antioxidant properties.
- It defends against cancer.
- It protects healthy hair and skin.

Vitamin B3

Vitamin B3 is also known as niacin. It is essential for the process of turning carbohydrates, fat, and alcohol into energy so that it can be used by the body. It helps with keeping the skin healthy. It also supports major systems of the body, including the nervous and digestive systems. Niacin is very stable when it is exposed to heat, so a very small portion of it loses its nutritional value during cooking.

Foods that are rich sources of niacin include meat, fish, poultry, milk, eggs, cereal, nuts, mushrooms, whole grain breads, and foods that contain a higher quantity of protein.

When consumed in large quantities, niacin leaves a drug-like effect on blood fats and nervous system. Side effects include getting flushed, itching, nausea, and a possibility of the liver getting severely damaged, even though positive changes are witnessed in the blood fats.

Symptoms of Vitamin B3 Deficiency

Niacin deficiency is called pellagra. It is common among people who consume large amounts of alcohol. It is also common in people whose diets consist exclusively of corn. Some other causes of pellagra are interlinked with problems in digestion, where the body is unable to absorb the niacin effectively. The primary symptoms of pellagra are known as the three Ds. These Ds are dementia, diarrhea, and dermatitis. Other noticeable symptoms of pellagra are inflammation and swelling of the tongue, irritability, loss of appetite, mental confusion, weakness, and dizziness. If not treated in due time, pellagra can lead to death.

There are multiple symptoms of pellagra. These include:

- Symmetrical lesions that appear on both sides of the body. The lesions are visible at pressure points on the body and areas of the skin that are most likely to be exposed to the sun. Some people develop lesions that cover their entire hands and/or feet.

- Butterfly-shaped lesions are formed on the face. They also form a shape that resembles a 'necklace' of lesions around the neck that develop after spending time in the sun.

- Pain, swelling, mouth irritation, or other mucous membranes in genitals, such as the vagina or the urethra. Severe deficiency can cause the tongue to turn red or even swell to a certain degree. Some people develop sores under the tongue or on their lips, which can cause irritation.

- Pain and burning sensations in the throat, chest, or stomach.

- There are digestive pains. These include swelling, vomiting, nausea, diarrhea, and constipation. Some individuals develop an ulcer in their bowels that results in bloody diarrhea, literally.

- Changes in personality and mental health, including losing contact with reality (psychosis), confusion, memory problems, depression, and paranoia.

Sometimes, these symptoms are incorrectly diagnosed as mental illness.

Sources of Vitamin B3

- Portobello mushroom
- Cooked potato
- Liver
- Cooked or canned tuna
- Soy burger
- Pumpkin seed
- Black-eyed pea
- 100 percent bran cereal
- Toasted wheat germ cereal
- Instant cooked oatmeal
- Cottage cheese
- Soya milk

Our body can convert an amino acid called tryptophan into Vitamin B3. Tryptophan-rich foods, such as turkey and eggs, contain numerous Vitamin B3 properties. So including these foods in the diet may help prevent Vitamin B3 deficiency.

Vitamin B5

Vitamin B5 is also known as pantothenic acid. It is essential because it helps with the metabolism of carbohydrates, proteins, fats, and alcohol that we consume. It is also beneficial in producing red blood cells in the body, as well as steroid hormones.

Foods that contain high quantities of pantothenic acid include liver, meat, milk, kidney, eggs, yeast, peanuts, and legumes. Vitamin B5 is also found in many other food items but these are the ones that are rich in pantothenic acid.

The deficiency of pantothenic acid is extremely rare and uncommon. The symptoms that point to the deficiency of pantothenic acid include loss of appetite, lack of proper sleep, constipation, fatigue, vomiting, and intestinal distress.

Pantothenic acid is taken as a medicine for diseases such as osteoarthritis, rheumatoid arthritis, Parkinson's disease, nerve pain, premenstrual syndrome (PMS), and for an enlarged prostate, among others. It is also taken for the treatment of physical and mental stress and anxiety. It is used for reducing signs of aging, lowering vulnerability to infections – such as cold among others, retarded growth, and shingles. It is also effective for the treatment of skin disorders, used for stimulating adrenal glands, chronic fatigue syndrome, salicylate toxicity, streptomycin neurotoxicity, dizziness, and wound healing.

Pantothenic acid can also be used as an applicant for external use in the form of dexpanthenol, which is made from it. It can be used for the treatment of itching on the skin, mild eczema, insect bites and stings, poison ivy, rashes from diapers, and general skin acne. It is also effective for treating skin reactions to radiation therapy.

Symptoms of Vitamin B5 Deficiency

The most common symptom of Vitamin B5 deficiency, which is also severely irritating, is burning foot syndrome. The person experiences a lack of feeling in their feet, accompanied by intense inflammatory pain in the leg. This also brings a constant feeling of fatigue and weakness that can be felt throughout the body. Other notable symptoms include insomnia, anemia, vomiting, contraction of muscles, and abnormal developments on the skin.

Sources of Vitamin B5

- Chicken liver
- Salmon
- Sunflower seed
- Sun-dried tomato
- Avocado
- Corn
- Broccoli
- Mushroom
- Yoghurt
- Cauliflower

There are plenty of other sources of Vitamin B5, including nutritional yeast. Nutritional yeast is considered to be an excellent source of Vitamin B for people who are vegetarians and vegans. Supplements, such as multivitamins, always contain this essential Vitamin.

The health benefits of Vitamin B5 include the alleviation of conditions such as asthma, hair loss, allergy, stress, anxiety, respiratory disorders, and heart problems. It also helps boost immunity, reduce osteoarthritis and signs of aging, increases resistance to various types of infections, stimulates physical growth, and helps manage diabetes and skin disorders.

Vitamin B5 is widely known to be beneficial in treating serious mental disorders, such as chronic stress and anxiety. A healthy diet should contain an appropriate amount of this Vitamin to ensure good health and proper functioning of all organ systems. It performs a wide variety of functions in our body. These include the fabrication of steroids and the extraction of fats and proteins, as well as the production of neurotransmitters in the brain.

To sum it up, the essence of Vitamin B5 affects every important aspect of our health that is possible. Vitamin B5:

- Helps with hormone stimulation
- Helps relieve stress
- Improves heart health
- Improves stamina
- Improves skin health
- Helps improve hair health
- Maintains immune system health
- Maintains hemoglobin count
- Increases metabolism
- Synthesizes cholesterol
- Heals wounds
- Prevents rheumatoid arthritis

Chapter 4

Vitamin B6

Vitamin B6 is also known as pyridoxine. It is one of the Vitamins that belongs in the Vitamin B complex family. All the Vitamins belonging to the B category, including Vitamin B6, play an important role in a variety of physical and psychological functions. They are commonly known for maintaining a healthy metabolism, nerve and liver function, healthy vision, overall health of the skin, and boosting energy levels in the body.

Vitamin B6 has several derivatives. These include pyridoxal, pyridoxal 5-phosphate, and pyridoxamine. They are all important compounds that are responsible for biological functions. Vitamin B6 is used by our body every single day because of its importance. It helps in carrying out major functions, including movement, memory, and energy expenditure, along with regular blood flow in the body. Therefore, a Vitamin B6 deficiency can show up in many different symptoms. Only some of these are temporary, others are more serious and long lasting.

Vitamin B6 helps the body maintain a healthy nervous system, besides helping it make hemoglobin that carries oxygen in red blood cells throughout the body. It helps in providing energy from the food that we eat, balances blood sugar levels, acts as a natural pain treatment to boost mood, and creates antibodies that our immune system uses to protect us. Vitamin B6 is clearly vital for our bodies.

A Vitamin B6 deficiency is a rarity in western developed nations, where most people acquire enough calories and aren't experiencing malnourishment. In fact, experts feel that some people actually consume high levels of this Vitamin.

The recommended amount of Vitamin B6 for an average adult who falls under the age of 50 is 1.3 milligrams. Normally, this amount is relatively easy to get from your diet, assuming you eat enough calories in general.

However, the intake recommendation jumps up as you get older. Experts recommend that adults over 50 get up to 1.7 milligrams daily. The increase in Vitamin B6 is needed as someone moves up in the age bracket. This makes older people more likely to experience a Vitamin B6 deficiency.

Symptoms of Vitamin B6 Deficiency

There are studies that have linked a Vitamin B6 deficiency with an increased risk for a range of different disorders and symptoms, even though a B6 deficiency is not very common.

A Vitamin B6 deficiency can cause symptoms over a period of time. These include:

- Mood swings, such as irritability, anxiety and depression
- Confusion and uncertainty
- Muscle pain
- Lower levels of energy or fatigue
- Worsening of PMS symptoms and anemia

Understand that Vitamin B6 is really important for nerve function. A Vitamin B6 deficiency is commonly linked with neuropsychiatric disorders, including seizures, migraines, chronic pain, and mood disorders like depression.

Other studies have indicated that lower levels of Vitamin B6 status is linked to an increased risk of heart disease and rheumatoid arthritis. Other researches show that Vitamin B6 deficiency is more common among older people, with the risk of Alzheimer's disease and other forms of dementia increasing as someone ages. Their level of Vitamin B6 decreases correspondingly in their bodies.

Since they are at a higher risk of having a Vitamin B6 deficiency, it's recommended that older people should have their Vitamin B6 levels tested by their doctor if they begin to experience a loss of appetite, extreme weight loss, and nutrient malabsorption for any reason.

Recommended Daily Amount of Vitamin B6

Vitamin B6 benefits can be found in many foods that are commonly eaten in our daily lives. These include nuts and seeds, certain kinds of meat and poultry, avocados, legumes and beans. Vitamin B6 also includes B complex Vitamins, as well as many multivitamins. Consuming these are especially beneficial if you experience a lot of stress, low energy levels, mood swings, a lot of physical activity, heart diseases, and symptoms relating to PMS, as well as chronic pain or regular migraines. These pertain to people who are above 50 years of age.

Depending on your age and gender, the recommended daily allowance for Vitamin B6 is as follows:

- Newborn-6 months: 0.3 milligrams
- Children 1-8 years: 0.5-0.6 milligrams
- Children 4-16 years: 0.6-1.0 milligrams
- Boys 14-18 years: 1.2-1.3 milligrams
- Men and women 19-50 years: 1.3 milligrams
- Men 51 years and older: 1.7 milligrams
- Women 51 years and older: 1.5 milligrams
- Pregnant women: 1.9 milligrams
- Breastfeeding women: 2.0 milligrams

All B Vitamins are water-soluble. This means that they will be flushed out of the body and will be dissolved in your urine if you ingest too much of them. This is the reason that there isn't much concern about overdosing on Vitamin B6 or reaching toxic levels. However, in rare instances, too much Vitamin B6 can cause some harmful reactions.

Consuming too much Vitamin B6 is usually a result of taking supplements and eating or drinking fortified processed foods that contain synthetic B Vitamins. These include fortified grain products and energy drinks. When someone has a higher level of Vitamin B6 within their body, the reactions include muscle numbness, confusion and other unpleasant temporary symptoms.

Sources of Vitamin B6

Vitamin B6 can be found in high levels naturally in several foods, including the following:

- Avocado
- Chicken Breast
- Blackstrap Molasses
- Turkey Breast

- Grass-Fed Beef
- Sunflower Seeds
- Sesame Seeds
- Garbanzo Beans
- Amaranth Grain
- Pistachio Nuts
- Tuna
- Pinto Beans

Taking Vitamin B6 Supplements

Since Vitamin B6 is water-soluble, the body is not able to store any leftover Vitamin B6 for future use. This also means that one must regularly eat foods that are rich with B Vitamins or take supplements to continue to meet the daily requirements.

While taking Vitamin B supplements can prove to be helpful for some people, it's always advised to get your nutrients from natural and fresh food sources. The body knows exactly what to do with the Vitamins that are naturally found in such food sources as opposed to synthetic nutrients that are added in fortified foods.

Vitamins are best used by the body to their full capacity. They are actually utilized as complex groups of molecules that interact and are dependent upon each other. Hence, you get the most benefits from Vitamin supplements when you consume them in the way nature intended for you to eat them.

If you are going to be taking any supplements that contain Vitamin B6, be sure to purchase a high-quality product that is made from real food sources and doesn't contain any artificial chemicals or toxins. High-quality Vitamin B complex supplements are made by joining different collaborative nutrients together so your body recognizes the Vitamins and minerals. The body can then use them in a natural way, giving you the most beneficial results.

Health Benefits of Vitamin B6

Maintains Healthy Blood Vessels

Vitamin B6 is required to regulate levels of a compound

called homocysteine that is present in blood. Homocysteine is a type of amino acid that is acquired from eating protein sources, especially certain kinds of meat. High levels of homocysteine in the blood results in inflammation and the formation of heart disease and diseases of the blood vessel, which may lead to a heart attack.

In the absence of Vitamin B6, homocysteine gathers in the body and damages blood vessel linings. This can set the stage for dangerous plaque buildup, which can lead to a heart attack or stroke.

Studies have shown that when patients take Vitamin B6 along with folate, total homocysteine concentrations are distinctly reduced. Vitamin B6 helps to treat high homocysteine levels so the body can heal the damage that is caused to blood vessels.

Vitamin B6 also plays a role in managing blood pressure and cholesterol levels. These two are other important factors for preventing heart disease.

Supports Brain Function

The B6 Vitamin benefits include helping in the proper

development of our brain and brain function. Studies have shown that a Vitamin B6 deficiency could have a negative effect on memory function and can contribute to cognitive impairment, Alzheimer's and dementia as someone ages. Other studies also link a Vitamin B6 deficiency to possibly be a prominent contributing factor to Alzheimer's disease.

One way Vitamin B6 impacts brain function is by controlling homocysteine levels, which are not only a risk factor in the case of heart diseases, but also cause damage to neurons of the central nervous system as well.

Vitamin B6 also plays an important role in making the hormones, serotonin and norepinephrine. These two hormones are known as "happy hormones" that help to control mood, energy and concentration. Researchers believe that certain behavior disorders in children, including ADHD, are caused by low serotonin levels and therefore, consuming Vitamin B6 might have a beneficial effect on children that suffer with these learning and behavioral disorders.

Helps with Mood Improvement

Some prescription antidepressant medications work the

same way that Vitamin B6 does, by raising levels of serotonin in the brain. Research has shown that Vitamin B6 has a significant impact on the central production of both serotonin and GABA (*gamma*-Aminobutyric acid) neurotransmitters in the brain. These important hormones control moods and are imperative for preventing depression, pain, fatigue and anxiety. Thus, Vitamin B6 has been associated with increasing mood and preventing mood disorders.

Because Vitamin B6 is involved in hormone production in the brain, it's believed to be effective in treating mood disorders and certain brain diseases that can develop as a result of deficiencies in neurotransmitter function. Research suggests that patients consuming Vitamin B6 supplements have their moods uplifted, experience less pain, and avoid having a lack of energy and focus.

Helps Reduce Anemia

Vitamin B6 is needed to create hemoglobin in the blood, which is transported by red blood cells throughout the body to help bring oxygen to cells and mobilize iron. Anemia develops when someone doesn't produce enough red blood cells. This results in symptoms including fatigue, pains and aches in the body, to name a few. Studies show that consuming plenty of Vitamin B6 can help lower symptoms of anemia and prevent it from occurring in certain cases.

Improves Eye Health

In many instances, a poor diet or nutrient deficiency are the underlying causes that lead to many eye diseases. Studies have shown that combining Vitamin B6 along with other Vitamins, including folate, can help with the prevention of eye disorders and loss of vision.

Vitamin B6 is believed to help slow the onset of certain eye diseases, including age-related macular degeneration.

Helps Prevent or Reduce Symptoms of Rheumatoid Arthritis

Low levels of Vitamin B6 have been associated with increased symptoms of rheumatoid arthritis (RA), including more severe kinds of pain. Certain early studies are discovering that people with RA may need more Vitamin B6 than other healthy people because they experience ongoing muscle aches and joint pains due to chronic inflammation. Vitamin B6 benefits include the soothing of pain and it can be useful in supplement form for controlling aches in the muscles and joints due to arthritis.

Helps Reduce High Blood Pressure

Some earlier studies suggest that taking Vitamin B6 supplements may be able to help lower blood pressure levels in people with the existing condition of high blood pressure. Vitamin B6 increases blood flow, lowers build up in the arteries and is important in the prevention of common factors that lead to heart diseases.

Helps Relieve Symptoms of Premenstrual Syndrome

Consuming plenty of Vitamin B6 or taking B complex Vitamins can be helpful in the prevention or treatment of PMS symptoms. Studies have shown that Vitamin B6 helps combat breast pain, nausea, cramps, fatigue, headaches and even particular kinds of acne that occur before a woman's menstrual cycle.

It's believed that Vitamin B6 helps with PMS because of its positive effects on neurotransmitters that are responsible for pain management in the brain. It also plays a key role in increasing blood flow and managing hormones. It's recommended for women who experience frequent PMS symptoms to take B complex Vitamins regularly, especially the 10 days before menstruating.

Helps Decrease Nausea During Pregnancy

Studies have found that taking Vitamin B6 is effective in relieving the severity of nausea and "morning sickness" that is common during pregnancy. A study showed that after patients tracked the severity of their nausea over 24 hours before treatment with Vitamin B6, and again afterwards, the group who took Vitamin B6 experienced a reduced level of nausea when compared with the other group that did not.

Helps Combat Asthma

Some studies have shown that Vitamin B6 benefits include decreasing the occurrence of asthma attacks. The nutrient has helped those who suffer with asthma to reduce symptoms of wheezing that are associated with asthma attacks, as well as lowering the severity and frequency of the attacks occurring.

Helps Regulate Sleep Cycles

Vitamin B6 helps the body produce melatonin, which is an important hormone that helps us fall asleep. Melatonin is responsible for allowing us to regulate our own internal clock so we know when it's time to wake up and consume the energy within, and also when it's time to unwind and fall asleep during the night.

Prevents Kidney Stone Development

Some studies show that taking Vitamin B6 along with other minerals, including magnesium, may be able to prevent or treat kidney stones. Vitamin B6 is usually helpful in doing this for patients who are at an increased risk of ending up with kidney stones that occur due to other illnesses.

Interactions of Vitamin B6

Vitamin B6 can interact with other medications when taken in high quantities. If you're being treated for any of the following conditions and are on medications, it's always a good idea to consult with your doctor before taking any supplements, including Vitamin B6.

Some medications that interact with Vitamin B6 include:

- Drugs used for treating Parkinson's and Alzheimer's disease, as well as anemia, seizures or heart disease.
- Any of the drugs that are used in chemotherapy.
- Cycloserine (Seromycin) or Isoniazid, used for treating tuberculosis.

- Hydralazine (Apresoline), used for treating high blood pressure.
- Penicillamine used to treat rheumatoid arthritis.
- Theophylline (TheoDur), used to treat asthma.
- Antibiotics including Tetracycline.
- Antidepressant medications including Pamelor, Elavil, desipramine, Norpramin and Tofranil.
- Some antidepressants called monoamine oxidase inhibitors (MAOIs) may also be able to reduce blood levels of Vitamin B6.

> # Chapter 5

Vitamin B9

Vitamin B9, also called folic acid, is a form of Vitamin that is water-soluble. It is a vital ingredient in the formation of the nucleic acids (DNA and RNA) that form part of all genetic material.

It is a Vitamin from Vitamin B complex that is quite similar to Vitamin B12. Vitamin B9 and its forms carry out the crucial functions of creating more red blood cells, preventing hearing loss, and preserving the brain health of infants.

Importance of Vitamin B9

Vitamin B-9 includes both folate and folic acid. These substances make it important for multiple functions in the body. According to the British Dietetic Association (BDA), folic acid is vital for producing red blood cells, as well as:

- the synthesis and repair of DNA and RNA
- assisting in rapid cell division and growth
- enhancing overall brain health
- Preventing old age-related hearing loss

There are many dietary requirements for a pregnant woman which can ensure that the baby's health is perfect when the baby is born. Consumption of these folic acids is one such dietary requirement. Folic acid helps in the prevention of the fetus developing major congenital deformities of the brain or spine. These include neural tube defects, such as spinal bifida and anencephaly.

Women who are planning to get pregnant should consume folic acid supplements for a full year before conceiving to reduce the risk of these developments. Folic acid is also considered to play a preventive role in a range of conditions.

Benefits of Vitamin B9

Folic acid, iron and calcium have long been considered the most essential elements for prenatal wellness. However, there are innumerable benefits of Vitamin B9 to support the overall health of the body.

Use of Vitamin B9 During and After Pregnancy

This is probably the top reason why the Vitamin is hugely popular among pregnant women. Folic acid is best known to prevent birth defects and ensures good spinal development of an unborn baby. If an expectant mother suffers from Vitamin B9 deficiency, it can lead to serious issues including neural tube defects.

If you're pregnant or plan to get pregnant anytime soon, it's extremely important to get enough folic acid in your body on a daily basis. Folic acid, as mentioned above, is the synthetic form of Vitamin B9. It is also known as folate.

Folic acid helps prevent NTDs (neural tube defects) in the body. These are serious birth defects of the spinal cord (such as spina bifida) and the brain (such as anencephaly). The neural tube is the part of the embryo that is responsible for your baby's spine and brain development. NTDs affect about 3,000 pregnancies annually in the United States.

Neural tube defects occur at a very early stage of development. Sometimes, even before many women know that they're pregnant. This is why it's important to begin taking folic acid before you start trying to conceive a baby.

The Centers for Disease Control and Prevention (CDC) report that women who take the recommended daily dose of folic acid, beginning at least one month before conception and during the first trimester of pregnancy, reduce their baby's risk of neural tube defects by up to 70 percent.

Some research suggests that folic acid may help in lowering the baby's risk of other defects as well. These include cleft lip, cleft palate, and certain types of heart defects. It may also reduce your risk of **preeclampsia**, a serious blood pressure disorder that affects about 5 percent of pregnant women.

Your body needs this nutrient to make normal red blood cells and prevent a type of anemia. It's also essential for the production, repair, and functioning of DNA, our genetic map and a basic building block of cells. Getting enough folic acid is particularly important for the placenta's rapid cell growth and your developing baby.

Prevents Premature Ageing

It is common for the skin to sag as we get old. However, research reveals that people who regularly consume folic acid can delay the onset of aging signs, such as wrinkles. Vitamin B9 supplementation also **delays aging** by preventing the production of stress hormones in the human body.

Moreover, Vitamin B9 also boosts the metabolism and promotes efficient absorption of nutrients. Thus, people who want to stay young forever must include good sources of folate in their diet or use a folic acid supplement.

Prevents Cardiac Arrests

Not many people know that excess of homocysteine, a kind of amino acid, leads to many heart complications. It can increase the risks of suffering a stroke at late stages in life. One of the most crucial benefits of Vitamin B9 is that it regulates the level of homocysteine in the body to support good heart health. In addition, folic acid also controls the level of deposition of cholesterol in the human heart, therefore preventing a large number of heart disorders.

Helps Maintain Good Mental Health

Another significant benefit of consuming Vitamin B9 is a successful treatment of many types of emotional disorders. This is why many doctors prescribe a folic acid supplement to relieve anxiety and depression.

Improves the Production of Red Blood Cells

Vitamin B9 is utilized in red blood cell production and maturation, and it supports the complex procedure of how our body produces blood cells.

Deficiency of this Vitamin can lead to a blood disorder known as megaloblastic anemia. This is a health complication where an individual does not have enough red blood cells, and the red blood cells they have are very large. This Vitamin is directly involved in generating red blood cells, which is called erythropoiesis, along with other B-Complex Vitamins.

Although Vitamins B9 aren't the only nutrients needed to produce red blood cells, it does play a crucial role in the process. Hence, it is a universal supplement to recommend for combination treatment anemia.

Helps Combat Depression

Folate has natural antidepressant properties. If you are feeling low for no reason, it could be due to low folate levels. This is because folate plays a vital part in the production of serotonin and dopamine (the 'feel good' hormones). Depression and anxiety are caused by an imbalance of both these important neurotransmitters.

Folic acid offers the same effects as many popular antidepressants. Vitamin B9 is immensely useful for relieving depression symptoms and lowering anxiety levels among patients. Folic acid also helps individuals who suffer from eating disorders.

It is common for women to experience hot flashes, post-menopause, due to estrogen deficiency and a disturbance in the thermoregulatory system. Folic acid is shown to increase estrogen levels and reverses depression symptoms in women after menopause.

Helps With Coenzyme Activity

Vitamin B9 is regarded as an important co-enzyme. This implies that it works efficiently with other enzymes to perform many crucial processes of the body, such as DNA synthesis.

Supports Muscle Build-up

If you are looking forward to a harmless way of building and supporting muscle tissues; Vitamin B9 supplementation is one of the best ways to ensure that you protect your muscles from the effects of daily wear and tear.

Combats Free Radicals

Folic acid works as an antioxidant to destroy free radicals in the body. In addition to Vitamin C and Vitamin E, this Vitamin is essential to help rid the body of free radicals that are actually byproducts of oxygen metabolism and lead to toxicity.

This damage can negatively affect the central nervous

system and lead to complications such as Alzheimer's and dementia. Moreover, this activity also results in many types of inflammatory diseases, as well as diabetes and hair loss.

When you regularly consume folic acid, the body successfully flushes out toxins from the body and keeps you safe from more than 20 diseases that are associated with free radicals in the body.

Prevents Cancer Development

Another remarkable benefit of folate is that it is crucial for the formation of nucleic acids and functions as a cofactor in the stability, repair and synthesis of DNA molecules. This is vital for controlling cell differentiation and the expression of genes. It is common for abnormalities to develop when DNA methylation is not controlled, eventually leading to cancer. The risks of developing many forms of cancers can be reduced by maintaining a regular consumption of Vitamin B9.

Boosts Fertility

Just like the folate helps in giving birth to healthy kids, the same technique applies to adult humans as well. It helps synthesize our DNA, and promotes the survival and development of the fetus. According to a study involving guinea pigs, researchers observed that having insufficient amounts of folic acid in our body, even for a temporary period of time, can lead to adverse consequences for our reproductive health.

Hence, you can enhance your fertilization level by consuming folic acid. Other conditions that can be improved by Vitamin B9 are:

Helps Prevent the Development of Autism

A recent study connected folic acid deficiency with autism. The investigators concluded, *"Preconception folic acid before conception and during early pregnancy may reduce autism spectrum disorder risk in those with inefficient folate metabolism."*

ALEX OSELU OWITI; B. PHARM, MT, M. PHARM, PHD

Helps Prevent the Development of Cleft Lip and Palate

A literature review carried out in 2014 concluded that consuming folic acid supplements might reduce the risk of a cleft palate.

Helps Prevent Rheumatoid Arthritis

Folic acid is often used to support a methotrexate prescription for rheumatoid arthritis.

Methotrexate is an effective medicine for this condition. However, it is also known to remove folate from the body. This can cause gastrointestinal symptoms in between 20 and 65 percent of people who use the drug.

However, folic acid supplements have been shown to reduce the gastrointestinal side effects of methotrexate by 79 percent. Speak to a doctor for recommendations on how much to take, and how often. 1 milligram (mg) per day is often prescribed.

Who Should Take Vitamin B9?

Folic acid helps protect the bones and brains of infants. All women who are pregnant or planning to become pregnant should consume more folic acid according to March of Dimes, a research organization focused on preventing deformity and death in newborn infants.

They also recommend that women take folic acid before getting pregnant, as well as during the first 4 weeks following conception.

Every woman capable of getting pregnant should be taking daily folic acid supplements. Women over the age of 14 years should take 400 micrograms (mcg) per day, and this should increase to 600 mcg during a pregnancy.

Women should maintain a daily intake of 500 mcg while they are lactating.

Women who take folic acid supplements for at least 12 months before becoming pregnant could reduce the risk of having a premature infant by over 50 percent.

The researchers concluded:

"Preconception folate supplementation is associated with a 50 to 70 percent reduction in the incidence of early spontaneous preterm birth."

Folic acid is essential for the growth of the spinal cord in the womb. It is important that an expectant mother consumes enough folic acid during the earliest stages of development. This is because the spinal cord is one of the first parts of the body to form in the womb.

Sources of Vitamin B9

Dark green vegetables are good sources of folic acid. Nonetheless, be careful not to overcook them as the folic acid content can drop considerably when exposed to heat.

The following foods are known to be rich in folic acid:

- Asparagus
- Baker's Yeast
- Broccoli
- Brussels Sprouts
- Cabbage
- Cauliflower
- Egg Yolk
- Jacket Potato
- Kidney
- Lentils

- Lettuce
- Liver (although, women should not consume this during pregnancy)
- Many Fruits, especially Papaya and Kiwi
- Milk
- Oranges
- Parsnips
- Peas
- Spinach
- Sunflower Seeds
- Whole-Wheat Bread, as it is usually fortified

Below is the chart according to portion size.

Foods	Portion Size	Folates*
Poultry offal, roasted or braised	100g (3.5oz)	345-770μg
Lamb and calf liver, sautéed	100g (3.5oz)	331-400μg
Legumes, cooked	100g (3.5oz)	229-368μg
Pork liver, braised or sautéed	100g (3.5oz)	100g (3.5oz)
Spinach, boiled	125ml (0.5 cup)	139μg
Asparagus, boiled	125ml (0.5 cup)	134μg
Enriched pasta, cooked	125ml (0.5 cup)	120-125μg
Flaxseed	60ml (0.25 cup)	108μg
Soybeans, boiled or sautéed	125ml (0.5 cup)	83-106μg
Broccoli, boiled	125ml (0.5 cup)	89μg
Romaine lettuce	250ml (1 cup)	64μg

Sunflower seeds, roasted	60ml (0.25 cup)	78μg
Sunflower seed butter	30ml (2 tbsp.)	78μg
Beets, cooked	125ml (0.5 cup)	72μg
Sprouted soybeans	125ml (0.5 cup)	64μg
Spinach, raw	250ml (1 cup)	61μg
Orange juice	125ml (0.5 cup)	58μg
Brussels sprouts, cooked	4 sprouts (80 g)	50μg
Okra (gumbo), boiled	125ml (0.5 cup)	39μg
Walnuts, hazelnuts and filberts, dehydrated, not blanched	60ml (0.25 cup)	33μg

It is always better to get nutrients from natural food sources rather than supplements. Seek out these food options and work them into your diet.

Symptoms of Vitamin B9 Deficiency

Folic acid deficiency occurs when not enough folate or folic acid is present in the body.

Aside from **anemia** and congenital deformities, folic acid deficiency can result in other health problems, including:

- A higher risk of developing clinical depression.

- Possible problems with memory and brain function.
- A higher risk of potentially developing allergic diseases.
- A higher potential long-term risk of lower bone density.

The *Medical Journal of Australia* advised in January 2011 that the prevalence of folate deficiency in the country had dropped considerably since the introduction of the compulsory fortification of wheat flour in bread making.

Anemia Caused by Folic Acid Deficiency

Having too little folate (Vitamin B9) in our blood causes folic acid deficiency anemia.

Folate is necessary for our body to make new red blood cells. Our body needs red blood cells to carry oxygen to our organs. Not having enough red blood cells causes a condition called anemia that can make you feel weak and tired.

Your baby may be at higher risk of developing serious birth defects like spina bifida if you have folic acid deficiency anemia during pregnancy. Spina bifida causes the baby's spinal column to be malformed.

If you're folic acid deficient, taking supplements to increase your folic acid level can reduce your risk of developing anemia. What's more, experts at Harvard Medical School say that getting enough folic acid can reduce the risk of developing colon cancer and heart disease. Individuals can develop folic acid deficiency anemia if they do not consume enough folic acid.

As folate is important for producing and maintaining red blood cells; inadequate levels can mean that there are not enough red blood cells to supply the body with a healthy level of oxygen. This condition can appear in people who require higher quantities of folate and are not taking supplements; such as women who are pregnant and lactating. Folic acid deficiency anemia can occur in people with underlying conditions, such as sickle cell anemia. It can also affect people with conditions that affect folate absorption. Alcohol abuse or kidney disease can reduce the ability of the body to effectively absorb folate.

Some medications, such as those used for treating rheumatoid arthritis, cancer, and seizures, may increase the risk of folic acid deficiency anemia.

Causes of Folic Acid Anemia

Malnutrition is the most common cause of folic acid deficiency anemia. Eating a diet low in Vitamins or overcooking foods can contribute to malnutrition. Heavy bleeding can also lead to anemia. Foods rich in folic acid include citrus fruits, leafy green vegetables, and fortified cereals. Some people have trouble absorbing folic acid from food.

Pregnancy

Pregnancy causes folic acid deficiency for several reasons. The body is slower in absorbing folic acid during pregnancy, and the fetus consumes our body's folic acid as it grows. Morning sickness that results in vomiting can cause you to lose folic acid.

Malabsorption

Malabsorption occurs when our body can't properly absorb a Vitamin or mineral. Diseases such as celiac disease and medications, including those to control seizures, can disrupt the way our body absorbs folic acid.

Diagnosis of Folic Acid Deficiency Anemia

Other blood conditions can cause symptoms similar to folic acid deficiency anemia. You'll need to see a doctor for a diagnosis. A doctor will do a complete blood count (CBC) test to determine if you have folic acid deficiency anemia. This test will reveal if your red blood cell count is low.

The doctor may also order a blood test to check your folic acid levels. This is called a red blood cell folate level test. If you're of childbearing age, your doctor may order a pregnancy test to determine if this is the cause of your deficiency. They'll also ask questions about your eating habits to see if malnutrition is the culprit.

Be sure to mention to the doctor whether or not you're taking any medications since some can contribute to folic acid deficiency.

Treatment of Folic Acid Deficiency Anemia

The goal of treatment is to increase our body's level of folic acid. The easiest way is to consume folic acid tablets on a daily basis until the deficiency is under control. However, you might need to receive folic acid intravenously if your levels are too low.

Along with taking supplements, you should eat foods that are high in folic acids, such as pinto beans, spinach, and oranges. Eat plenty of fresh foods and avoid processed or fried foods. They're usually low in nutrients and high in fat.

Harvard Medical School guidelines recommend consuming 400 mcg (micrograms) of folic acid per day. Pregnancy and certain health conditions may warrant taking more. The most you can take without developing symptoms of an overdose is 1,000 mcg of folic acid per day.

Side Effects of Vitamin B9

There are no serious side effects when taking folic acid. In some rare cases, individuals report an **upset stomach**. Even if a person takes more folate than needed, there is no cause for concern. As folic acid is water-soluble, any excess will be naturally passed out in the urine.

Chapter 6

Vitamin B12

Vitamin B12 is a water-soluble Vitamin, like all the other B Vitamins. This means it can dissolve in water and travel through the bloodstream. The human body can store Vitamin B12 for a timespan of three to five years. Any excess or unwanted Vitamin B12 is flushed out from the body through excretion in the urine.

Vitamin B12 is the largest and most structurally complicated of all the Vitamins. It occurs naturally in meat and seafood products and can only be industrially produced through the process of bacterial fermentation synthesis. Vitamin B12 assists your body with producing DNA and red blood cells. It supports your immune system, and encourages healthy nerve function.

ALEX OSELU OWITI; B. PHARM, MT, M. PHARM, PHD

Sources of Vitamin B12

For a healthy body, it is of utmost importance that you consume your Vitamin B's. Although it's pretty easy to get most B Vitamins by eating and maintaining a balanced diet containing lots of fresh produce and whole grains, Vitamin B12 is another story. It is found naturally in animal sources only. That means people who don't eat meat or dairy, vegans or vegetarians, can have trouble reaching the daily recommended 2.4 mcg (micrograms) dose of Vitamin B12.

It is different for different people. For example, the requirement is 2.6 mcg for pregnant women and 2.8 mcg if you're a breastfeeding mother. People who suffer from digestive problems and issues like celiac disease and adults older than the age of 50 years are also at a higher risk of being deficient due to absorption problems, which can cause weakness, fatigue, and lightheadedness. But most often you will be on your way to a B12-rich diet if you eat at least some of these 15 foods.

They are as follows:

Clams

Best Ways to Eat Them

Clams are delicious in pasta dishes or stews. Steam them until the shells crack open, or boil for about five minutes till the shells have opened.

Oysters

Other Body Benefits

Oysters contain more zinc than any other food. A large 32 mg in six raw oysters is 400% of your RDA, the essential mineral that supports your immune system by helping fight off colds. Zinc can encourage testosterone production, which may improve libido and is helpful in keeping women's ovaries healthy.

Best Ways to Eat Them

Enjoy oysters as an appetizer or in a seafood stew.

Mussels

Other Body Benefits

In addition to Vitamin B12, mussels are also a good source of protein, potassium, Vitamin C, and omega-3 fatty acids.

Best Ways to Eat Them

Steam them as an appetizer, or serve in a seafood stew.

Crab

Other Body Benefits

Crab meat contains Vitamins A, B, and C, as well as magnesium. Just like oysters, they're full of zinc. A can of blue crab meat has 4.7 mg, or 58% of your RDA.

Best Ways to Eat It

Prepare crab cakes as an appetizer, add crabmeat to seafood chowder, or mix into your salad.

Sardines

Other Body Benefits

You may be surprised to learn that these tiny fishes are packed with calcium. Just 3 ounces of sardines have the same amount as 8 ounces of milk. Sardines also contain Vitamin D and omega-3 fatty acids. If you buy them canned in oil, be sure to rinse them before cooking to get rid of excess salt.

Best Ways to Eat Them

Sardines are great in a marinara sauce over spaghetti squash. Toss in any leftover veggies you have in the fridge to give the sauce a nutritional kick.

Trout

Other Body Benefits

Trout is one of the fatty fishes. It is a great source of Vitamin D and omega-3 fatty acids. They promote healthy brain function and fight inflammation.

Best Ways to Eat It

Trout is great when grilled with a little extra virgin olive oil and served alongside garlic-sautéed spinach or even a baked sweet potato.

Salmon

Other Body Benefits

Like trout, salmon is a rich source of protein and heart healthy omega-3 fatty acids. Also good: One 3-ounce salmon fillet contains more than 100% of your DV of Vitamin D.

Best Ways to Eat It

To maximize salmon's many health benefits, experts recommend baking it in the oven or grilling it instead of eating it fried, dried, or salted. It is best when served with some vegetables.

Tuna

Other Body Benefits

Tuna is loaded with Vitamin D. A 3-ounce serving contains about 150 IUs, or 25% DV. Like salmon and trout, it's also a rich source of omega-3 fatty acids, including eicosapentaenoic acids (EPAs) and docosahexaenoic acids (DHAs), which are considered to help in lifting spirits.

Best Ways to Eat It

When buying it canned, it is best to go for one with chunky light tuna in water. And if you're adding it into a salad, it is suggested to leave out the mayonnaise.

Haddock

Other Body Benefits

Though it contains fewer omega-3 fatty acids than oilier fishes, such as salmon, haddock is still an amazing low-fat protein source. It's also a healthier option if you're worried about mercury since it has a lesser level of the chemical than other fish. These include tuna, halibut, and cod.

Best Ways to Eat It

Bake haddock in the oven with simple seasonings, such as lemon and fresh herbs. Or grill the fillets and serve on a bun as a healthier alternative to a regular cheese burger.

Beef

Other Body Benefits

Beef is another great source of zinc. It contains 7 mg in 3 ounces. Also packed with protein and the B Vitamin riboflavin, which is considered to help alleviate PMS symptoms.

Best Ways to Eat It

Combine beef with veggies, whole grains, and good fats, such as ginger. Stir fry it with beef over brown rice. It is advised to eat it in moderation since red meat has a high level of cholesterol, and consuming too much could increase your risk of heart disease.

Milk

Other Body Benefits

Not only is it a good source of calcium and Vitamin D, but milk might also help some women tackle PMS symptoms. Whole milk could offer additional benefits. Studies show that women who consumed more than one serving of high-fat dairy on a daily basis were 25% less likely to experience ovulation problems than those who did not.

Best Ways to Eat It

Try making a smoothie with milk, frozen fruit, almond butter, ginger, and cinnamon.

Yogurt

Other Body Benefits

Yogurt is a great source of calcium, magnesium, and protein. Studies show that consuming it regularly could prevent diabetes and prevent high blood pressure. Yogurt is also a great digestive aid, balancing the microflora in your gut and easing IBS symptoms because of the probiotics.

Best Ways to Eat It

It is best when incorporated into smoothies or mixed with oats, fruit, nuts, and herbs, such as fresh mint.

Eggs

Other Body Benefits

Eggs are a great source of protein and Vitamin D, which is important for helping your body absorb calcium and maintain strong bones.

Best Ways to Eat It

Hard-boiled, soft-boiled, poached, or scrambled eggs. If you're watching your cholesterol, keep an eye on portion sizes: one egg yolk contains about 60% of your daily allotment of dietary cholesterol.

Chicken

Other Body Benefits

Chicken is a lean protein, making it a terrific fat-burning food. It has a high thermogenic effect, which means your body can burn about 30% of the calories it contains by digestion only.

Best Ways to Eat It

There are countless healthy ways to eat chicken; grilled, roasted, or baked in the oven.

Turkey

Other Body Benefits

Just one serving of lean turkey has nearly half your RDA of selenium. Selenium is a trace mineral that supports immune function. Turkey contains tryptophan, which is a chemical that assists with sound sleep.

Best Ways to Eat It

Oven roasted turkey breast on a garden salad with sprouts and potatoes, or any other vegetable of your choice.

Choose white turkey meat and try to skip the skin because it contains more saturated fat.

Benefits

Vitamin B12 is crucial to the normal function of the brain and the nervous system. It is also involved in the formation of red blood cells and helps to create and regulate DNA. The metabolism of every cell in the body depends on Vitamin B12 as it plays a part in the synthesis of fatty acids and energy production. Vitamin B12 enables the release of energy by helping the human body absorb folic acid.

The human body produces millions of red blood cells with every passing minute. These cells cannot multiply properly without Vitamin B12. The production of red blood cells drops if Vitamin B12 levels are too low. Anemia can occur if the red blood cell count decreases exponentially.

Intake requirements

In the USA, the National Institutes of Health (NIH) recommend that teens and adults over the age of 14 years should consume a 2.4 micrograms (mcg) of Vitamin B12 a day. Pregnant women should be sure to consume 2.6 mcg, and lactating women should intake 2.8 mcg. Excessive intake of Vitamin B12 has not demonstrated toxic or harmful qualities. However, people are always advised to consult with their doctors and physicians before choosing to take supplements.

Some medications may interact with Vitamin B12. These include metformin, proton pump inhibitors, and h2 receptor agonists. They are often used for peptic ulcer disease. All of these drugs may interfere with Vitamin B12 absorption in our bodies. The antibiotic chloramphenicol, or chloromycetin, may also interfere with red blood cell production in people who regularly take supplements.

Who Is At Risk of Vitamin B12 Deficiency

Vegans face a risk of Vitamin B12 deficiency, as their diet excludes animal-sourced food products. Pregnancy and breastfeeding can worsen its deficiency in vegans. Plant-sourced foods and plant based diets do not have enough cobalamin to guarantee long-term health.

People with pernicious anemia may lack Vitamin B12. Pernicious anemia is an autoimmune disease that has a negative impact on the blood. Patients with this disorder do not have enough intrinsic factor (IF), which is a protein in the stomach that allows the body to absorb Vitamin B12.

Other at-risk groups include people with small intestine problems, such as an individual whose small intestine has been surgically shortened. They may not be able to absorb cobalamin properly. People suffering with Crohn's disease may be at risk, too.

Gastritis, celiac disease, and inflammatory bowel disease may lead to a deficiency because these conditions cause improper absorption of nutrients and can also be reduced.

People with chronic alcoholism may lack Vitamin B12 since their bodies are also not able to absorb nutrients as required.

Individuals treating diabetes with metformin are advised to monitor their levels of Vitamin B12 since it can reduce the absorption of Vitamin B12.

Treatment includes Vitamin B12 injections. A Vitamin B12 injection must be administered to people that have problems with nutrient absorption only, and not general patients or without proper consultation.

Supplements of Vitamin B12

Some people have difficulties absorbing Vitamin B12 from food sources and may need to take supplements. These include older adults, patients with pernicious anemia, and those with achlorhydria, or intestinal disorders, who may have problems absorbing Vitamin B12 from food.

Supplements can be consumed orally or in a nasal spray. However, oral supplements do not help in many deficiency cases. In these circumstances, Vitamin B12 may be injected.

Vegans can take supplements to avoid a deficiency, as the vegan diet removes the meat products that are a natural source of the Vitamin. This is particularly important during pregnancy and while breastfeeding.

Side Effects of Vitamin B12

The side effects of taking Vitamin B12 are very limited.

It is not considered to be toxic in high quantities, and even 1000 mcg doses are not considered to be harmful.

Cyanocobalamin is an injectable form of the supplement that contains traces of cyanide, which is a substance containing poisonous properties. As a result, some concerns have been raised about its possible effects. However, many fruits and vegetables contain these traces, and they are not considered to have a significant health risk.

This type of supplement is not, however, recommended for people suffering from kidney disease.

9 Signs and Symptoms of Vitamin B12 Deficiency

It plays an essential role in the production of your red blood cells and DNA, as well as the proper functioning of your nervous system.

Vitamin B12 is naturally found in animal foods, including meats, fish, poultry, eggs and dairy. However, it can also be found in products fortified with B12, such as some varieties of bread and plant-based milk.

Unfortunately, B12 deficiency is common, especially in elderly people. You're at risk of deficiency if you don't get enough from your diet or aren't able to absorb enough from the food you eat.

People at risk of a B12 deficiency include:

- The elderly.
- Those who've had surgery that removes the part of the bowel that absorbs B12.
- People on the drug metformin for diabetes.
- People following a strict vegan diet.
- Those taking long-term antacid drugs for heartburn.

Unfortunately, symptoms of a Vitamin B12 deficiency can take years to show up, and diagnosing it can be complex. A B12 deficiency can sometimes be mistaken for a folate deficiency.

Low levels of B12 cause your folate levels to drop. However, if you have a B12 deficiency, correcting low folate levels may simply mask the deficiency and fail to fix the underlying problem.

Here are 9 signs and symptoms of a Vitamin B12 deficiency:

ALEX OSELU OWITI; B. PHARM, MT, M. PHARM, PHD

Pale or Jaundiced Skin

People with a B12 deficiency often look pale or have a slight yellow tinge to the skin and whites of the eyes, a condition known as jaundice. This happens when a lack of B12 causes problems with your body's red blood cell production.

Vitamin B12 plays an essential role in the production of the DNA that are needed to make red blood cells. Without it, the instructions for building the cells are incomplete, and cells are unable to divide.

This causes a type of anemia called megaloblastic anemia, in which the red blood cells produced in your bone marrow are large and fragile.

These cells are too large to pass out of your bone marrow and into your blood circulation stream. Therefore, you don't have as many red blood cells circulating around your body, and your skin can appear to look pale in color.

The fragility of these cells also means that many of them break down, causing an excess of bilirubin. Bilirubin is a slightly red or brown-colored substance, which is produced by the liver when it breaks down old blood cells. Large amounts of bilirubin are what give your skin and eyes a yellow tinge.

Weakness and Fatigue

Weakness and fatigue are common symptoms of Vitamin B12 deficiency. They occur because your body doesn't have enough Vitamin B12 to make red blood cells that can carry oxygen throughout your body.

As a result, you are unable to efficiently transport oxygen to your body's cells, making you feel tired and weak.

In the elderly, this type of anemia is often caused by an autoimmune condition known as pernicious anemia.

People with pernicious anemia don't produce enough of an important protein called intrinsic factor. Intrinsic factor is essential for preventing a B12 deficiency, as it binds with Vitamin B12 in your gut: helping with proper absorption.

Sensations of Pins and Needles

One of the more serious side effects of a long-term B12 deficiency is nerve damage. This can happen over time, as Vitamin B12 is an important contributor to the metabolic pathway that produces the fatty substance, myelin. Myelin surrounds your nerves as a type of protection and insulation. Without B12, myelin is produced differently, and your nervous system isn't able to function properly.

One common sign of this happening is paresthesia, which can be best described as the sensation of pins and needles; a prickling sensation in your hands and feet.

Interestingly, the neurological symptoms associated with B12 deficiency usually occur alongside anemia. However, one study found that about 28% of people had neurological symptoms of B12 deficiency, without any signs of anemia. That being said, sensations of pins and needles are a common symptom that can have many causes, so this symptom alone is not particularly a sign of B12 deficiency.

Changes to Mobility

If left untreated, the damage to your nervous system caused by a B12 deficiency could cause changes to the way you walk and move around.

It may even affect your balance and coordination, making you more prone to falling.

This symptom is often seen in undiagnosed B12 deficiency in the elderly people since individuals over the age of 60 are more likely to have a B12 deficiency. However, preventing or treating deficiencies in this group may improve mobility.

Also, this symptom may be present in young people who have a severe, untreated deficiency.

Glossitis and Mouth Ulcers

Glossitis is a term used to describe an inflamed tongue. If you have glossitis, your tongue changes color and shape, making it painful, red and swollen.

The inflammation can also make your tongue look smooth, as all the tiny bumps on your tongue that contain your taste buds stretch out and vanish. As well as being painful, glossitis can change the way you eat and speak.

Studies have shown that a swollen and inflamed tongue that has long straight lesions on it could be an early sign of Vitamin B12 deficiency.

Additionally, some people with a B12 deficiency may experience other oral symptoms, such as mouth ulcers, paresthesia in the tongue or a burning and itching sensation in the mouth.

Breathlessness and Dizziness

If you become anemic due to a B12 deficiency, you may feel you're usually out of breath and a bit dizzy, especially when you overexert yourself. This is because your body lacks the red blood cells it needs to get enough oxygen to your body's cells.

Disturbed Vision

One symptom of Vitamin B12 deficiency is blurred or disturbed vision. This can occur when an untreated B12 deficiency results in damage to the nervous system and to the optic nerve that leads to your eyes.

The damage can disrupt the nervous signal that moves from your eye to your brain, affecting your vision. This condition is known as optic neuropathy. Although a matter of concern, it is treatable by supplementing with B12.

Mood Swings and Changes

People with B12 deficiency often report changes in mood. In fact, low levels of B12 have been linked to mood and brain disorders like depression and dementia.

The *"homocysteine hypothesis of depression"* has been suggested as a potential explanation for this link. This theory suggests that high levels of homocysteine caused by low levels of B12 could cause damage to the brain tissue and interfere with signals to and from your brain, leading to mood changes and severe mood swings.

Some studies suggest that in certain people who are deficient in B12, supplementing it with the Vitamin can reverse signs.

If you have a deficiency, taking a supplement may help improve your mood. However, it's not a substitute for other proven medical therapies in the treatment of depression or dementia, since there can also be other reasons and causes for those.

High Temperature

A very rare but occasional symptom of B12 deficiency is a high temperature. It's not clear why this occurs, but some doctors have reported cases of fever that has normalized after treatment with low levels of Vitamin B12. However, it's important to keep in mind that high temperatures are more commonly caused by illness, not a B12 deficiency.

Chapter 7

Vitamin C

Vitamin C is also known as L-ascorbic acid, ascorbic acid, or L-ascorbate. Vitamin C is a vital nutrient for our health. It helps in the formation and maintenance of red blood cells, bones, skin, and blood vessels. It occurs naturally in some foods, especially fruits and vegetables. Supplements containing Vitamin C are also available. Humans are unable to synthesize Vitamin C endogenously, so it is an essential dietary component that must be incorporated into our daily food intake.

Vitamin C is known for biosynthetic and antioxidant functions. It plays an important role in immune function and helps in the improvement of nonheme iron absorption, the form of iron present in plant-based foods. Insufficient Vitamin C intake causes scurvy, which is identified and bracketed by fatigue or lassitude, widespread weakness of connective tissue, and capillary fragility.

ALEX OSELU OWITI; B. PHARM, MT, M. PHARM, PHD

Importance of Vitamin C

A few excellent sources of Vitamin C are fruits, green vegetables, and vitamin supplements.

Vitamins, including Vitamin C, are organic compounds. An organic compound is one that exists in living things. It contains the elements carbon and oxygen.

Vitamin C is water-soluble, and the body does not store it. To maintain adequate levels of Vitamin C, humans need a daily intake of food that are rich with Vitamin C.

Vitamin C plays an important role in a number of bodily functions, including the production of collagen, L-carnitine, and some neurotransmitters. It helps metabolize proteins and its antioxidant activity can be helpful in reducing the risk of some cancers.

Collagen, which Vitamin C helps to produce, is the main component of connective tissue and the most abundant protein in mammals. Between 1 and 2 percent of muscle tissue is made of collagen. It is a vital component in fibrous (made of fibers) tissues such as:

- Tendons
- Ligaments
- Skin
- Cornea
- Cartilage
- Bones
- Blood Vessels
- Gut

In the case of wound healing, research as long ago as 1942 suggested that wounds took longer to heal if someone was suffering from scurvy.

Scurvy is a disease that results from Vitamin C deficiency. Its symptoms include swollen joints, bleeding gums and loose teeth, anemia, and tiredness.

Rebound scurvy can happen if a person takes very high doses of Vitamin C and then discontinues it abruptly.

ALEX OSELU OWITI; B. PHARM, MT, M. PHARM, PHD

Wound Healing, Infections, and Tuberculosis

Research has established that wounds, cuts, and grazes may heal faster in people whose diets contain adequate quantities of Vitamin C, more than the quantity that is usually available from a normal diet. This may be because Vitamin C contributes to collagen production which in turn accelerates wound healing.

Vitamin C, as an antioxidant, also helps in repairing tissues and reduces damage from inflammation and oxidation.

People with adequate levels of Vitamin C are much able to fight off infections as compared to people who have a Vitamin C deficiency in their systems. Vitamin C may also help prevent acute respiratory infections, especially in cases of malnutrition and people who are physically stressed.

Researchers have also found that Vitamin C can kill drug-resistant tuberculosis (TB) bacteria in a laboratory culture. A study published in 2013 suggests that adding Vitamin C to TB drugs could shorten the time span that it would take for therapy.

Vitamin C Prevents Cancer Development

Vitamin C may help in treating cancer. As an antioxidant, it protects the body against oxidative stress and helps in the prevention of oxidation of other molecules. It appears to reproduce other antioxidants in the body. Studies suggest that Vitamin C may complement chemotherapy for cancer patients.

Oxidation reactions produce free radicals. Free radicals can trigger reactions that damage cells. Adequate doses of Vitamin C have been found to reduce the speed of growth of some types of cancerous tissues. Researchers have proposed using Vitamin C in cancer patients whose treatment options are limited.

More studies are needed to understand which cancers could be affected by Vitamin C and which other effective treatments can be used in conjunction with Vitamin C, as well as the long-term effects of this approach.

Some scientists have disputed the use of Vitamin C in cancer treatment. A number of doctors support it and are already using it in treatment.

The United States Food and Drug Administration (FDA) has not yet approved the use of Vitamin C in the treatment of cancer patients, including those who are undergoing chemotherapy and radiation therapy. Furthermore, it is not recognized as a treatment.

Other benefits of Vitamin C may include the following:

- Smokers and people with a compromised immune system may benefit from Vitamin C supplements.
- Cardiovascular health: Vitamin C may widen the blood vessels, and this could help protect against heart diseases and hypertension, or even aid with reducing high blood pressure.
- Cholesterol levels: These were found to be lower in individuals with steady levels of Vitamin C.
- Cataracts: Vitamin C may help in lowering the risk of cataracts, as well as of age-related macular degeneration.

- Diabetes: Patients are less likely to experience deterioration of the kidneys, eyes, and nerves if they eat plenty of fruits and vegetables that are rich in Vitamin C.

- Anemia: Vitamin C enhances the absorption of iron.

- Lead: Levels may be reduced if there is an adequate intake of Vitamin C.

- Histamine: This is a substance that is produced by the immune system. It results in inflammation and other problems. A 1992 study found lower blood levels of histamine in people who took 2 grams (g) of Vitamin C per day.

- Seasickness: A group of 70 people who took either 2g of Vitamin C or a placebo, then spent 20 minutes on a life raft in a wave pool, had reduced levels of seasickness.

Vitamin C Prevents Common Cold

Vitamin C can strengthen the body's immune system

which gives the body the capability to fight off infectious and pathogenic microorganisms such as the virus that cause common cold and other viral or bacterial infections. Furthermore, adequate doses of Vitamin C may help with protection against the effects of severe physical activity and cold temperatures. People with low Vitamin C, because of smoking or old age, for example, may find supplements beneficial.

Sources and Requirements of Vitamin C

Adult males should consume 90 milligrams (mg) of Vitamin C per day and females should consume 75 mg per day according to the National Institutes of Health (NIH). During pregnancy, women should have 85 mg a day, and 120 mg while breastfeeding. Consuming red peppers and other vegetables and fruits should provide enough Vitamin C for most people.

The best sources of Vitamin C are fresh fruits and vegetables. Heating and cooking in water can destroy some of the Vitamin C content, so raw foods are best since the Vitamin C properties remain intact.

Sources of Vitamin C

Foods containing Vitamin C include:

- Red pepper
- Orange juice
- Orange
- Grapefruit juice
- Kiwi fruit
- Green pepper
- Broccoli
- Tomato juice
- Cantaloupe
- Cabbage
- Cauliflower
- Potato
- Tomato
- Spinach
- Green peas

The people at risk of Vitamin C deficiency include:

- Smokers and passive smokers.
- People who have a limited food variety in their diet.
- Infants who consume evaporated or boiled milk.

- People with malabsorption and a few chronic diseases.

Smokers have lower levels of Vitamin C than nonsmokers, partly because they have higher levels of oxidative stress. Smoking also causes inflammation and damage to the mucous membranes of the mouth, throat, and lungs.

Vitamin C is necessary for healthy mucosa and reducing inflammation, so the NIH recommends that smokers consume an extra 35 mg of Vitamin C each day compared to people who don't smoke.

Side Effects of Vitamin C

Too much Vitamin C is unlikely to cause a problem in your body. However, a high intake of over 1,000 mg of Vitamin C a day may mean that not all the Vitamin C is absorbed in the intestine. This can lead to complications such as diarrhea and gastrointestinal discomfort.

A high intake of Vitamin C through supplements, rather than through diet, may result in kidney stones. It may increase the risk of cardiovascular problems in women after menopause, but this is not proven yet.

People with hereditary hemochromatosis, which is an iron absorption disorder, should consult their doctor before taking Vitamin C supplements, as high Vitamin C levels could lead to tissue damage. The maximum recommended daily intake of Vitamin C for adult males and females is 2,000 mg.

Medicinal Value of Vitamin C

- Vitamin C deficiency.
- Taking Vitamin C by mouth or injecting as a shot prevents and treats Vitamin C deficiency, including scurvy.
- Also, taking Vitamin C can reverse problems associated with scurvy.

Other Effects of Vitamin C

- Iron absorption: Administering Vitamin C along

with iron can increase how much iron the body absorbs in adults and children.

- A genetic disorder in newborns called tyrosinemia: Taking Vitamin C by mouth or as a shot improves a genetic disorder in newborns, in which blood levels of the amino acid tyrosine are too high.

- Age-related vision loss (age-related macular degeneration, AMD): Taking Vitamin C, Vitamin E, beta-carotene, and zinc helps prevent AMD from becoming worse in people at high risk for developing advanced AMD. It's too soon to know if the combination helps people at lower risk for developing advanced AMD. Also, it's too soon to know if Vitamin C helps prevent AMD.

- Increasing protein in the urine (albuminuria): Taking Vitamin C plus Vitamin E can reduce protein in the urine in people with diabetes.

- Irregular heartbeat (atrial fibrillation): Taking Vitamin C before and for a few days after heart surgery helps prevent irregular heartbeat after heart surgery.

- Emptying the colon before a colonoscopy: Before a person undergoes a colonoscopy, the person must make sure that their colon is empty. This emptying is called bowel preparation. Some bowel preparation involves drinking 4 liters of medicated fluid. If Vitamin C is included in the medicated fluid, the person only needs to drink 2 liters. This makes people more likely to follow through with the emptying procedure. Also, fewer side effects occur. A specific medicated fluid containing Vitamin C (MoviPrep, Salix Pharmaceuticals, Inc.) has been approved by the U.S. Food and Drug Administration (FDA) for bowel preparation.

- Common cold: There is some controversy about the effectiveness of Vitamin C for treating the common cold. However, most research shows that taking 1-3 grams of Vitamin C might shorten the course of the cold by 1 to 1.5 days. Overall however, Vitamin C does not appear to prevent colds.

- Chronic pain condition called complex regional pain syndrome: Taking Vitamin C after surgery or injury to the arm or leg seems to prevent complex regional pain syndrome from developing.

- Redness (erythema) after cosmetic skin procedures: Using a skin cream containing Vitamin C might decrease skin redness following laser resurfacing for scar and wrinkle removal.

- Upper airway infections caused by heavy exercise: Using Vitamin C before heavy physical exercise, such as a marathon, might prevent upper airway infections that can occur after heavy exercise.

- Stomach inflammation (gastritis): Some medicine used to treat H. pylori infection can worsen stomach inflammation. Taking Vitamin C along with one of these medicines called omeprazole might decrease this side effect.

- Gout: Higher intake of Vitamin C from the diet is linked to a lower risk of gout in men. But Vitamin C doesn't help treat gout.

- Worsening of stomach inflammation caused by medicine used to treat Pylori infection: Some medicine used to treat H. pylori infection can worsen stomach inflammation. Taking Vitamin C along with one of these medicines, called omeprazole, might decrease this side effect.

- Abnormal breakdown of red blood cells (hemolytic anemia): Taking Vitamin C supplements might help manage anemia in people undergoing dialysis.

- High blood pressure: Taking Vitamin C along with medicine to lower blood pressure helps lower systolic blood pressure (the top number in a blood pressure reading) by a small amount. But it does not seem to lower diastolic pressure (the bottom number). Taking Vitamin C does not seem to lower blood pressure when taken without medicine to lower blood pressure.

- High cholesterol: Taking Vitamin C might reduce low-density lipoprotein (LDL or "bad") cholesterol in people with high cholesterol.

- Lead poisoning: Consuming Vitamin C in the diet seems to lower blood levels of lead.

- Helping medicines used for chest pain work longer: In some people who take medicines for chest pain, the body develops tolerance and the medicines stop working as well. Taking Vitamin C seems to help these medicines, such as nitroglycerine, retain their effects for longer.

- Osteoarthritis: Taking Vitamin C from dietary sources or from calcium ascorbate supplements seems to prevent cartilage loss and worsening of symptoms in people with osteoarthritis.

- Physical performance: Eating more Vitamin C as part of the diet might improve physical performance and muscle strength in older people. Also, taking Vitamin C supplements might improve oxygen intake during exercise in teenage boys. However, taking Vitamin C with Vitamin E does not seem to improve muscle strength in older men also doing a strength training program.

- Sunburn: Taking Vitamin C by mouth or applying it to the skin along with Vitamin E might prevent sunburn. But taking Vitamin C alone does not prevent sunburn.

- Wrinkled skin: Skin creams containing Vitamin C seem to improve the appearance of wrinkled skin.

Conditions Vitamin C is Ineffective For

- Bronchitis: Taking Vitamin C by mouth does not seem to have any effect on bronchitis.
- Asthma: Some people with asthma have low Vitamin C levels in their blood. But taking Vitamin C does not seem to reduce the chance of getting asthma or improve asthma symptoms in people who already have asthma.
- Hardening of the arteries (atherosclerosis): Higher intake of Vitamin C as part of the diet is not linked with a reduced risk of atherosclerosis. Also, taking Vitamin C supplements does not seem to prevent atherosclerosis from becoming worse in most people with this condition.
- Bladder cancer: Taking Vitamin C supplements does not seem to prevent bladder cancer or reduce bladder cancer-related deaths in men.
- Colon cancer: Higher intake of Vitamin C from food or supplements is not linked with a lower risk of cancer in the colon or rectum.
- Fracture: Taking Vitamin C does not seem to improve function, symptoms, or healing rates in people with a wrist fracture.

- Ulcers caused by a bacterium called Helicobacter pylori (H. pylori): Taking Vitamin C along with medicines used to treat H. pylori infection doesn't seem to get rid of H. pylori better than taking the medicines alone.

- Inherited nerve damage (hereditary motor and sensory neuropathy): Charcot-Marie-Tooth disease is a group of inherited disorders that cause nerve damage. Taking Vitamin C does not seem to prevent nerve damage from becoming worse in people with this condition.

- Eye damage associated with a medicine called interferon: Taking Vitamin C by mouth does not seem to prevent eye damage in people receiving interferon therapy for liver disease.

- Leukemia. Taking Vitamin C does not seem to prevent leukemia, or death due to leukemia, in men.

- Lung cancer: Taking Vitamin C, alone or with Vitamin E, does not seem to prevent lung cancer or death due to lung cancer.

- Melanoma: Taking Vitamin C, alone or with Vitamin E, does not prevent melanoma or death due to melanoma.

- Overall risk of death: High blood levels of Vitamin C have been linked with a reduced risk of death from any cause. But taking Vitamin C supplements along with other antioxidants does not seem to prevent death in and of itself.
- Pancreatic cancer: Taking Vitamin C together with beta-carotene, plus Vitamin E, does not prevent pancreatic cancer.
- High blood pressure during pregnancy (pre-eclampsia): Most research shows that taking Vitamin C with Vitamin E does not prevent high blood pressure during pregnancy.
- Prostate cancer: Taking Vitamin C supplements does not seem to prevent prostate cancer.
- Skin problems related to radiation cancer treatments: Applying a Vitamin C solution to the skin does not prevent skin problems caused by radiation treatments.

Insufficient Evidence

- Hay fever: Using nasal spray containing Vitamin C

seems to improve nasal symptoms in people with allergies that last throughout the year. Taking Vitamin C by mouth might block histamine in people with seasonal allergies. It has varying results.

- Alzheimer's disease: Higher intake of Vitamin C from food is linked with a reduced risk of Alzheimer's disease.

- Amyotrophic lateral sclerosis (ALS, Lou Gehrig's disease): Higher intake of Vitamin C from food or supplements is not linked with a reduced risk of ALS.

- Stomach damage caused by aspirin: Taking Vitamin C might prevent stomach damage caused by aspirin.

- Condition associated with an increased risk for developing allergic reactions (atopic disease): Higher intake of Vitamin C is not linked with a lower risk of eczema, wheezing, food allergies, or allergic sensitization.

- Attention deficit-hyperactivity disorder (ADHD): Taking high doses of Vitamins, including Vitamin C, does not seem to reduce ADHD symptoms. But taking lower doses of Vitamin C, along with flaxseed oil, might improve some symptoms, such as restlessness and self-control.

- Autism: Early research shows that taking Vitamin C might reduce the severity of autism symptoms in children.

- Breast cancer: It's too soon to know if higher intake of Vitamin C from food helps prevent breast cancer from developing. But a higher intake of Vitamin C from food seems to be linked with a reduced risk of death in people diagnosed with breast cancer. Also, taking Vitamin C supplements after being diagnosed with breast cancer seems to help reduce the risk of dying from breast cancer.

- Burns: Early research suggests that receiving a Vitamin C infusion within the first 24 hours of severe burns reduces wound swelling.

- Cancer: Higher intake of Vitamin C from food is linked with a lower risk of developing cancer. But taking Vitamin C supplements doesn't seem to prevent cancer. In people diagnosed with advanced cancer, taking large doses (10 grams) of Vitamin C by mouth doesn't seem to improve survival or prevent cancer from getting worse. But high doses of Vitamin

C might increase survival when given by IV.

- Hardening of the arteries after heart transplant: Early research shows that taking Vitamin C and Vitamin E for a year after a heart transplant helps prevent the hardening of arteries.

- Heart disease: Research on the use of Vitamin C for heart disease is controversial. More research on the use of Vitamin C supplements for preventing heart disease is needed. But increasing intake of Vitamin C from food might provide some benefits.

- Cataracts: Higher intake of Vitamin C from food is linked with a lower risk of developing cataracts. Some early research shows that people who take supplements containing Vitamin C for at least 10 years have a lower risk of developing cataracts. But taking supplements containing Vitamin C for less time doesn't seem to help.

- Cervical cancer: Some early research suggests that taking Vitamin C reduces the risk of cervical cancer.

- Side effects caused by chemotherapy: Early research suggests that higher intake of Vitamin C from food is linked with fewer chemotherapy side effects in children being treated for leukemia.

Precautions While Taking Vitamin C

Vitamin C is safe for most people when taken by mouth in recommended doses, when applied to the skin, when injected into the muscle, and when injected intravenously (by IV) by a doctor. In some people, Vitamin C might cause nausea, vomiting, heartburn, stomach cramps, headache, and other side effects. The chance of getting these side effects increases the more Vitamin C you take. Amounts higher than 2000 mg daily are POSSIBLY UNSAFE and may cause a lot of side effects, including kidney stones and severe diarrhea. In people who have had a kidney stone, amounts greater than 1000 mg daily greatly increase the risk of a kidney stone recurrence.

Special Precautions & Warnings

Pregnancy and breast-feeding: Vitamin C is LIKELY SAFE for women when taken orally in amounts no greater than 2000 mg daily, by subjects who are over the age of 19 years-old. 1800 mg every day is safe for girls who fall between 14 to 18 years-old, or when given intravenously (by IV), or intramuscularly and appropriately. Taking too much Vitamin C during pregnancy can cause problems for the newborn baby. Vitamin C is POSSIBLY UNSAFE when taken by mouth in excessive amounts.

Infants and children: Vitamin C is LIKELY SAFE when taken by mouth appropriately. Vitamin C is POSSIBLY UNSAFE when taken by mouth in amounts higher than 400 mg daily for children 1 to 3 years, 650 mg daily for children 4 to 8 years, 1200 mg daily for children 9 to 13 years, and 1800 mg daily for adolescents 14 to 18 years.

Alcoholism: Alcohol intake can cause the body to excrete Vitamin C in the urine. People who regularly use alcohol, especially those who have other illnesses, often have Vitamin C deficiency. These people might need to be treated for a longer time than normal to restore Vitamin C levels to normal.

Alzheimer's disease: Taking Vitamin C along with Vitamin E and alpha-lipoic acid might worsen mental function in people with Alzheimer's disease.

Angioplasty, a heart procedure: Avoid taking supplements containing Vitamin C or other antioxidant

Vitamins (beta-carotene, Vitamin E) immediately before and following angioplasty without the supervision of a health care professional. These Vitamins seem to interfere with proper healing.

Weight loss surgery: Weight loss surgery can cause the body to absorb more oxalate from food. This can increase the amount of oxalate in the urine. Too much oxalate in the urine can lead to problems, such as kidney stones. Vitamin C can also increase the amount of oxalate in the urine. Taking large amounts of Vitamin C after weight loss surgery might increase the risk of having large quantities of oxalate in the urine.

Cancer: Cancerous cells collect high concentrations of Vitamin C. Until more is known, only use high doses of Vitamin C under the direction of your oncologist.

Kidney disease: Vitamin C can increase the amount of oxalate in the urine. Too much oxalate in the urine can increase the risk of kidney failure in people with kidney disease.

Diabetes: Vitamin C might raise blood sugar. In older women with diabetes, Vitamin C in amounts greater than 300 mg per day increases the risk of death from heart disease. Do not take Vitamin C in doses greater than those found in basic multivitamins.

Metabolic deficiency called *"glucose-6-phosphate dehydrogenase"* (G6PD) deficiency: Large amounts of Vitamin C can cause red blood cells to break in people with this condition. Avoid excessive amounts of Vitamin C.

Blood-iron disorders, including conditions called *"thalassemia"* and *"hemochromatosis"*: Vitamin C can rapidly increase iron absorption, which might deteriorate the already worse conditions. Avoid large amounts of Vitamin C.

Kidney stones, or a history of kidney stones: Large amounts of Vitamin C can increase the chance of getting kidney stones. Do not take Vitamin C in amounts greater than those found in basic multivitamins, or those prescribed by your doctor.

Heart attack: Vitamin C levels are reduced during a heart attack. However, low Vitamin C has not been linked to a factor that would lead to an increased risk for heart attack.

Kidney transplant rejection: Long-term use of Vitamin C in high doses before a kidney transplant may elevate the risk of transplant rejection, or delay how long it takes until the transplanted kidney begins to function.

Schizophrenia: Taking Vitamin C, when paired with Vitamin E, might worsen psychosis in some people with schizophrenia when taken with antipsychotic drugs.

Sickle cell disease: Vitamin C might cause the condition to worsen. Avoid consuming large amounts of Vitamin C in this case.

Smoking and chewing tobacco: Smoking and chewing tobacco lowers Vitamin C levels in the body. Vitamin C intake in the diet should be increased in people who smoke or chew tobacco on a regular basis.

ALEX OSELU OWITI; B. PHARM, MT, M. PHARM, PHD

Chapter 8

Vitamin D

Vitamin D is produced by the body as a response to sun exposure. It can also be consumed in food or supplements. It is also known as the sunshine Vitamin. Having enough Vitamin D in the body is important for various reasons, including maintaining healthy bones and teeth. It may also protect against a series of conditions such as cancer, Type 1 diabetes, and multiple sclerosis. Despite the name, Vitamin D is considered a pro-hormone and not actually a Vitamin.

Vitamins are nutrients that cannot be created by the body and therefore must be taken in through our diet. However, Vitamin D can be synthesized by our body when sunlight hits our skin. It is said that adequate sun exposure on bare skin for 5-10 minutes, 2-3 times per week, allows most people to produce sufficient Vitamin D. But Vitamin D breaks down quickly, meaning that stores can run low, especially in winter. Recent studies have suggested that a substantial percentage of the global population is Vitamin D deficient.

Vitamin D has multiple roles in the body, helping to:
- Regulate insulin levels and aid diabetes management.
- Support lung function and cardiovascular health.
- Influence the expression of genes involved in cancer development.
- Maintain the health of bones and teeth.
- Support the health of the immune system, brain, and nervous system.

Health Benefits of Vitamin D

Healthier Bones

Vitamin D plays a substantial role in the regulation of calcium and maintenance of phosphorus levels in the blood, two factors that are extremely important for maintaining healthy bones. We need Vitamin D to absorb calcium in the intestines and to reclaim calcium that would otherwise be excreted through the kidneys. Vitamin D deficiency in children can cause rickets, a disease characterized by a severely bow-legged appearance due to softening of the bones.

In adults, Vitamin D deficiency manifests as osteomalacia, the softening of the bones, or osteoporosis. Osteomalacia results in poor bone density and muscular weakness. Osteoporosis is the most common bone disease among post-menopausal women, as well as older men.

Reduces the Risk of Flu

Children given 1,200 International Units of Vitamin D per day for a period of 4 months during the winter season recorded a drop in the risk of influenza by over 40 percent.

Reduces the Risk of Diabetes

Several observational studies have shown an inverse relationship between blood concentrations of Vitamin D in the body and a risk of type 2 diabetes. In people with type 2 diabetes, insufficient Vitamin D levels may negatively affect insulin secretion and glucose tolerance. In one particular study, infants who consume 2,000 International Units per day of Vitamin D had an 88 percent lower risk of developing type 1 diabetes by the age of 32.

Improves Infant Health

Children with normal blood pressure who were given 2,000 International Units (IU) per day had significantly lower arterial wall stiffness after 16 weeks, compared with children who were given only 400 IU per day.

Low Vitamin D status has also been associated with a higher risk and severity of atopic childhood diseases and allergic diseases, including asthma, atopic dermatitis, and eczema. Vitamin D may enhance the anti-inflammatory effects of glucocorticoids, making it potentially useful as a supportive therapy for people with steroid-resistant asthma.

Helps Maintain Healthy Pregnancy

Pregnant women who are deficient in Vitamin D seem to be at greater risk of developing preeclampsia and needing a cesarean section. Poor Vitamin D status is associated with gestational diabetes mellitus and bacterial vaginosis in pregnant women. It is also important to note that high Vitamin D levels during pregnancy were associated with an increased risk of food allergy in the child during their first two years of life.

Helps With Cancer Prevention

Vitamin D is extremely important for regulating cell growth and for cell-to-cell communication. Some studies have suggested that calcitriol (the hormonally active form of Vitamin D) can reduce cancer progression by slowing the growth and development of new blood vessels in cancerous tissue, increasing cancer cell death, and reducing cell proliferation and metastases. Vitamin D influences more than 200 human genes, which could be impaired when we do not have enough Vitamin D.

Vitamin D deficiency has also been associated with an increased risk of cardiovascular disease, hypertension, multiple sclerosis, autism, Alzheimer's disease, rheumatoid arthritis, asthma severity, and swine flu. However, more reliable studies are needed before these associations can be proven. Many of these benefits occur through Vitamin D's positive effect on the immune system's recommended intake of Vitamin D. Vitamin D intake can be measured in two ways: in micrograms (mcg) and International Units (IU).

One microgram of Vitamin D is equal to 40 IU of Vitamin D.

The recommended intakes of Vitamin D throughout life were updated by the U.S. Institute of Medicine (IOM) in 2010, and are currently set at:

- Infants 0-12 months - 400 IU (10 mcg).
- Children 1-18 years - 600 IU (15 mcg).
- Adults to age 70 - 600 IU (15 mcg).
- Adults over 70 - 800 IU (20 mcg).
- Pregnant or lactating women - 600 IU (15 mcg).

Vitamin D Deficiency

Although the body can create Vitamin D, there are many reasons because of which a deficiency can occur. For instance, darker skin color and the use of sunscreen reduce the body's ability to absorb the ultraviolet radiation B (UVB) rays from the sun needed to produce Vitamin D.

A sunscreen with sun protection factor (SPF) 30 can reduce the body's ability to synthesize the Vitamin by 95 percent. To start producing Vitamin D, the skin has to be directly exposed to sunlight and not covered by clothing.

People who live in northern latitudes or areas of high pollution, work at night and stay home during the day, or are homebound, should aim to consume extra Vitamin D from food sources whenever possible. Infants who are exclusively breast-fed need a Vitamin D supplement, especially if they are dark-skinned or have minimal sun exposure. The American Academy of Pediatrics recommends that all breastfed infants should get 400 IU per day of an oral Vitamin D supplement. Drops made specifically for babies are available for this purpose.

Although Vitamin D supplements can be taken, it is best to obtain any Vitamin or mineral through natural sources wherever possible.

Symptoms of Vitamin D Deficiency

Symptoms of Vitamin D deficiency may include:

- Impaired wound healing
- Fatigue
- Hair loss
- Muscle pain
- Getting sick or infected more often
- Painful bones and back
- Depressed mood

If Vitamin D deficiency continues for long periods of time, it can lead to conditions like:

- Depression
- Fibromyalgia
- Chronic fatigue syndrome
- Osteoporosis
- Obesity
- Diabetes
- Hypertension

- Neurodegenerative diseases, such as Alzheimer's disease

Vitamin D deficiency may also contribute to the development of certain cancers. These include breast, prostate, and colon cancers.

Causes of Vitamin D

Vitamin D deficiency can occur for a number of reasons:

- You don't consume the ideal quantities of Vitamin over time: This is likely if you follow a strict vegan diet, because most of the natural sources are animal-based, including fish and fish oils, egg yolks, fortified milk, and beef liver.
- You have dark skin: The pigment melanin reduces the skin's ability to make Vitamin D in response to sunlight exposure. Some studies show that older adults with darker skin are at high risk of Vitamin D deficiency.
- Your kidneys cannot convert Vitamin D to its active

form: As people age, their kidneys are less capable of converting Vitamin D to its active form, thus increasing their risk of Vitamin D deficiency.

- Your exposure to sunlight is limited: Because the body makes Vitamin D when your skin is exposed to sunlight, you may be at risk of deficiency if you are homebound, live in northern latitudes, wear long robes or head coverings for religious reasons, or have an occupation that prevents sun exposure.

- Your digestive tract cannot adequately absorb Vitamin D: Certain medical problems, including Crohn's disease, cystic fibrosis, and celiac disease, can affect your intestine's ability to absorb Vitamin D from the food you eat.

- You are obese: Vitamin D is extracted from the blood by fat cells, altering its release into the circulation. People with a body mass index of 30 or greater often have low blood levels of Vitamin D.

Tests for Vitamin D Deficiency

The most accurate way to measure how much Vitamin D

is in your body is the 25-hydroxy Vitamin D blood test. A level of 20 Nanograms/milliliters to 50 ng/ml is considered adequate for healthy people. A level less than 12 ng/ml indicates Vitamin D deficiency.

Treatment for Vitamin D Deficiency

Treatment for Vitamin D deficiency involves getting more Vitamin D through diet and **supplements**. Although there is no consensus on Vitamin D levels required for optimal health and it likely differs depending on age and health conditions, a concentration of less than 20 nanograms per milliliter is generally considered inadequate, requiring treatment.

Guidelines from the Institute of Medicine increased the recommended dietary allowance (RDA) of Vitamin D to 600 international units (IU) for everyone aged 1-70, and raised it to 800 IU for adults older than age 70 to optimize bone health. The safe upper limit was also raised to 4,000 IU. Doctors may prescribe more than 4,000 IU to correct a Vitamin D deficiency.

If you don't spend much time in the sun or always cover

your skin (**sunscreen** inhibits Vitamin D production), you should speak to your doctor about taking a Vitamin D supplement, particularly if you have risk factors for Vitamin D deficiency.

Sources of Vitamin D

Sunlight is the most common and efficient source of Vitamin D. The richest food sources of Vitamin D are fish oils and fatty fish. Here is a list of foods with that are rich in Vitamin D:

- Fortified skim milk
- Sardines, canned
- Tuna, canned
- Egg, chicken
- Cod liver oil
- Herring
- Swordfish
- Raw maitake mushrooms
- Salmon
- Orange juice

ALEX OSELU OWITI; B. PHARM, MT, M. PHARM, PHD

Vitamin D is unique, because it can be obtained from food *and* sun exposure. However, up to 50% of the world's population may not get enough sunlight, and 40% of people in the US are deficient in Vitamin D. This is partly because people spend more time indoors, wear sunblock outside and eat a Western diet low in good sources of this Vitamin.

The Reference Daily Intake (RDI) is 400 IU of Vitamin D per day from foods, but many health organizations recommend getting 600 IU. If you don't get enough sunlight, it should probably be closer to 1,000 IU per day.

Side Effects of Vitamin D

The Upper Level limit recommended for Vitamin D is 4,000 IU per day. However, the National Institutes of Health (NIH) has suggested that Vitamin D toxicity is unlikely at daily intakes below 10,000 IU per day.

Excessive consumption of Vitamin D, called hypervitaminosis D, can lead to over-calcification of bones. It can also cause hardening of blood vessels, kidney, lungs, and the heart. The most common symptoms of hypervitaminosis D are headache and nausea, but it can also include loss of appetite or parched mouth – which may sometimes lead to a metallic taste, vomiting, as well as constipation, and diarrhea.

It is best to get your required Vitamin D from natural sources. When choosing supplements, choose your brand carefully as the FDA does not monitor safety or purity of supplements. If you want to buy Vitamin D supplements, then there are genuine sources with thousands of customer reviews.

It is the total diet or overall eating pattern that is most important in prevention from diseases and achieving good health. It is better to eat a diet with a variety than to concentrate on one particular nutrient as the key to good health.

ALEX OSELU OWITI; B. PHARM, MT, M. PHARM, PHD

Chapter 9

Vitamin E

In this chapter, we discuss Vitamin E, and why doctors recommend the intake of this Vitamin. The importance of this Vitamin is also discussed along with its popularity as an antioxidant.

Vitamin E that occurs naturally exists in eight different forms, i.e. alpha, beta, gamma, and delta-tocopherol, and alpha, beta, gamma, and delta-tocotrienol. Each of these have varying levels of biological activity. However, the only form of Vitamin E that is recognized to meet human requirements is alpha-tocopherol.

Vitamin E belongs to the fat-soluble category of Vitamins. Like many other Vitamins, Vitamin E also has antioxidant properties that prevent free comprehensive damage to particular fats in the body that are important for health and also help in slowing down the ageing process. Vitamin E also helps in protecting the cells from damages caused by free radicals.

The compounds that are formed when our body breaks down the food that we eat and converts it into energy are known as free radicals. We are also exposed to these free radicals from our environment, such as from air pollution, cigarette smoking, and from the ultraviolet light that is released by the sun. Vitamin E is important for the proper functioning of a number of our organs, along with enzymatic activities and neurological processes.

Vitamin E is cannot be created by our bodies, therefore they must be taken from food sources. Although they are taken in very small amounts, which is enough for human bodies, their deficiency can cause several diseases.

Our body needs Vitamin E for various reasons. For example, it helps in boosting the immune system so that our body can fight against the invading bacteria and viruses. It also helps in widening the blood vessels so that the flow of blood is not interrupted from blood clotting. The cells in our body also use Vitamin E to communicate with each other and to carry out important functions.

The digestion of Vitamin E takes place in our small intestine by passive diffusion, while there is bile and dietary fat present. It is then transported through the lymph and bloodstream, and into the liver. Here, it is incorporated into very low-density lipoproteins so that they can be delivered to the tissues in the body.

The place where more than 90 percent of excess Vitamin E, in a non-esterified form, is stored is known as adipose tissues. The intake of Vitamin E needs to be monitored carefully as high intake apparently reduces its absorption rate in the body.

Health Benefits of Vitamin E

The key for a strong immune system and healthy eyes and skin is Vitamin E. Recently, the supplements of Vitamin E have become popular among people as antioxidants. Although deficiency of Vitamin E is very rare, people still take supplements in the hopes of preventing several diseases.

Improves and Regulates Menstrual Cycle

Vitamin E is found to have some properties that help in reducing the pain that women feel during their menstruation. Studies show that taking 200 IU of Vitamin E twice in one day, during menstrual period, helps in reducing the pain. It has also been shown to reduce pain and blood loss.

Improved Neurological Function

Research shows that Vitamin E plays a role in improving and maintaining neurological functions. The neurological functions of people, who have Vitamin E deficiency, can be improved a great deal by administering doses of Vitamin E. Omega 3 fatty acids are found in the brain, and Vitamin E plays a key role because of its antioxidant effects in protecting the membranes for oxidation and in saving the omega 3 fatty acids from peroxidation.

Helps Moisturize Skin

It is also found in moisturizers for men, because it treats

dry and skin flaking. People use Vitamin E in many different forms, such as in moisturizers, as explained above, and in the form of oil. They apply oil that is rich in Vitamin E in order to moisturize their skin and keep it from drying out.

Improves Wound Healing Ability

Although there is very limited research on the subject, some researchers suggest that supplements of Vitamin E can help in healing a wound. The reason why they believe this is because Vitamin E has properties that help cells in many ways. There is a lack of study in this regard, but nevertheless people are convinced that Vitamin E gives their body better healing ability.

Prevents Skin Cancer

There was a study conducted in 2003 on mice. The researchers in the study provided mice with supplements that contained Vitamin E. The results of their study revealed that the mice that were given doses of supplements of Vitamin E were less likely to develop skin cancer. This result was considered to be true even when these mice were exposed to ultraviolet light in large quantities. The supporters of Vitamin E oil and supplements used the results of this study to back their claim that Vitamin E helped in the prevention of skin cancer. However, the studies that were done on humans did not reveal any such benefits of Vitamin E.

Reduces Itching of Skin

Vitamin E does not provide a treatment for allergic reactions and infections, nor for other issues that are related to the itching of the skin. What happens is that Vitamin E moisturizes the skin, which offers a temporary relief from the itching that is caused by the dryness of the skin. When a person keeps their skin moisturized, they keep themselves safe from the itching of the skin. However, it can also be provided by any kind of oil and moisturizer, whether they contain Vitamin E or not. So, this benefit is debatable, and does not have enough scientific evidence to prove that it treats such allergic reactions or infections.

Alleviates Eczema

ALEX OSELU OWITI; B. PHARM, MT, M. PHARM, PHD

The flaking, itching, and dryness of skin that is associated with atopic dermatitis or eczema may be alleviated with the use of Vitamin E. Researchers have found that Vitamin E supplements could bring about significant improvements in the symptoms associated with eczema. Although there is a lack in the study of Vitamin E oil and its treatment of eczema, it may still increase the effectiveness of topical moisturizers.

Reduces Psoriasis

There was a study conducted that showed that topical Vitamin E can help in the reduction of symptoms related to psoriasis. It also revealed that there were no serious side effects of consuming Vitamin E. Though in comparison to the treatments of psoriasis that are available Vitamin E was not as effective, it is still a good option for people who want to avoid taking medications and who are suffering from mild psoriasis.

Applications of Vitamin E

There are several applications of Vitamin E, and people use it for far more complex reasons of their own. As we have already established that Vitamin E helps in the widening of the blood vessels, some people also use it for the prevention and treatment of heart disease and other symptoms related to the blood vessels such as high blood pressure, pain in the leg due to blocked arteries, chest pain, heart attack, and hardening of the arteries.

People also use Vitamin E for the treatment of diabetes and the complications that are associated with diabetes. As discussed earlier, people use it because they believe that it can prevent cancer -- particularly oral and lung cancer in people who smoke cigarettes, pancreatic cancer, prostate cancer, colorectal cancer, and polyps and gastric cancer.

Some people even use Vitamin E for diseases that are related to the nervous system and the brain. This includes, but is not limited to, dementias, night cramps, Parkinson's disease, epilepsy and restless leg syndrome. They do not use Vitamin E on its own, but they use it with other medications that are prescribed by doctors. Vitamin E is also used for disorders that involve the muscles and nerves.

Women in particular use Vitamin E for the prevention of the complications that arise with late pregnancy because of high blood pressure, painful periods, premenstrual syndrome, breast cysts, hot flashes associated with breast cancer, and menopausal syndrome.

At times, people also use Vitamin E in order to reduce the effects of some medical treatments, such as radiation and dialysis. Others use Vitamin E in order to reduce the harmful and unwanted effects of some medications, such as hair loss in people who are taking doxorubicin as well as lung damage in people who are taking amiodarone.

Additionally, people use Vitamin E to improve their physical endurance, for improving the strength of their muscles, for reducing the damage that is done to the muscles after exercise, and to increase their energy.

People use Vitamin E in different forms. Some take it in the form of supplements, and others use it in the form of oil, while others simply apply it on their skins. They do so in order to keep their skin from early aging, and to protect their skin from the harmful effects of chemicals that are used in the therapy of cancer.

Sources of Vitamin E

There are several sources from which a person can absorb Vitamin E into their body. We have already discussed Vitamin E in the form of products like moisturizers, oils, and supplements. Here, we will look at the natural sources of Vitamin E.

It can be obtained by consuming certain types of foods such as:

- Vegetable oils: These include soybean oil, corn, safflower, sunflower oil and wheat germ.
- Nuts: Such as filberts or hazelnuts, peanuts, pine nuts, brazil nuts and almonds.
- Seeds: For example, sunflower seeds.
- Green leafy vegetables: Like broccoli and spinach.
- Fortified breakfast cereals: Here, fortified means that the manufacturers have added Vitamins to their food products.
- Fruit juices
- Margarine
- Spreads
- Mamey Sapote: A species of tree that is native to Central America, Cuba, Costa Rica, and Mexico.

- Abalone: They are a type of gastropod shellfish.
- Goose Meat
- Atlantic Salmon
- Avocado
- Rainbow Trout: A type of fish.
- Mango
- Kiwi Fruit

Doses of Vitamin E

For the people who are above the age of 14 years, the recommended dietary allowance (RDA) for Vitamin E is 15 mg or 22.4 IU, as described by the National Institute of Health (NIH). For those women who are breastfeeding their infants, the RDA is 19 mg or 28.4 IU. For the purpose of safety, the recommended consumption limit of Vitamin E is 1000 mg or 1500 IU.

Most people around the world get their share of Vitamin E, in enough quantity to sustain their bodies, by eating a healthy diet. They do not necessarily need supplements for Vitamin E. In fact, it is recommended that you consult a doctor before taking any kind of supplements of Vitamin E, especially if you are on any kind of medications. There are several drugs in the market that do react with Vitamin E, and this reaction can worsen without warning or even without showing any symptoms.

Overdose of Vitamin E

Nothing over its limit can be healthy for the human body, and the same goes for Vitamin E. Although it can be acquired naturally, the consideration that is given to it should be the same as that given to any medical drug. The problem is that Vitamin E is fat-soluble, as explained earlier in this chapter, which is why excessive consumption of Vitamin E is not removed from the body through the urinary tract. It is stored in the body for later use, meaning that it can accumulate over time.

Symptoms of Vitamin E Deficiency

Early findings of Vitamin E deficiency have included symptoms such as abnormal cognition, night blindness, distal muscle weakness, decreased vibratory senses, decreased proprioception, and hyperreflexia. A continued deficiency of Vitamin E can lead to an increase in neurologic symptoms, and such patients can develop diffuse muscle weakness.

As we can see, there are several benefits and sources of Vitamin E. On the contrary, excessive use and intake can lead to diseases, and can cause several problems in the human body. So, it is best to consume Vitamin E by eating natural foods that contain Vitamin E, instead of going for Vitamin E supplements.

Chapter 10

Vitamin K

Throughout the book, we studied Vitamins, their sources, their nutritional value, the types of Vitamins, and their numerous benefits. However, in this chapter we will explore Vitamin K and its importance in blood coagulation. It also helps regulate the blood flow, which aids in the preventing blood loss.

Furthermore, it strengthens the bones. This lessens the risk of a fracture. Vitamin K belongs to the fat-soluble category of Vitamins. It plays an important role in reducing blood clotting, as well as metabolism of bones. It also helps in regulating the level of calcium in the blood.

Our body requires Vitamin K to make a clotting factor called prothrombin, which helps in the clotting of blood and our bone metabolism. People who use medications that reduce the blood viscosity, i.e. blood thinners, should consult their doctors before they consume Vitamin K.

Unlike other Vitamins, Vitamin K cannot be used as a dietary supplement. It actually exist in different forms, and the most important forms are Vitamin K1 and K2. Vitamin K1 can be obtained from green vegetables that are leafy, and some non-green leafy vegetables as well. On the other hand, Vitamin K2 is a group of compounds that are usually found in eggs, cheese, and meat. K2 is synthesized by bacteria, which is one of the reasons why Vitamin K1 is the most common and main form of Vitamin K that is available. Some people even use Vitamin K to treat osteoporosis and bone loss caused by steroids. However, there is very limited research in this regard.

Importance of Vitamin K

If the levels of Vitamin K in the human body are below their standard level, it can lead to uncontrolled and excessive bleeding. The deficiency of Vitamin K deficiency disorder is very rare, but it may be common among infants. One injection of Vitamin K is considered the standard treatment for infants. It is also used as a counter-dose for anything that cause excessive blood thinning effects.

Vitamin K deficiency is not common. But a person can be at a higher risk for Vitamin K deficiency if they are suffering from a disease that affects Vitamin K absorption in their digestive system. Other reasons that may provoke Vitamin K deficiency could be if the person is taking certain medications, is severely malnourished, or if they are alcoholic. In such extreme cases, it might be recommended to take Vitamin K medications as prescribed by the physician. Research has revealed that Vitamin K can also be used in the treatment of cancer, for the symptoms of morning sickness, for removal of spider veins, and for many other conditions, however more research is needed to confirm these facts.

Uses of Vitamin K

Vitamin K1 can be obtained from plants. After consumption, it is converted into its storage form, Vitamin K2, by the bacteria that are present in the large intestine. The small intestine absorbs Vitamin K2 and stores it in the fatty tissues and the liver.

Without the help from Vitamin K, our body cannot

produce prothrombin, which is a clotting factor that is essential for bone metabolism and blood clotting.

Vitamin K is effective for treating an inherited bleeding disorder called the Vitamin K dependent clotting factor deficiency (VKCFD). Individuals who are suffering from VKCFD can take Vitamin K by injection or orally in order to prevent bleeding as prescribed by the physicians.

Sources of Vitamin K

There are various foods that can be consumed in order to obtain Vitamin K. Some foods that are rich with Vitamin K include leafy green vegetables, such as kale or Swiss chard. It can also be obtained from vegetable oils and fruits. Foods that have Vitamin K1 include parsley, collard greens, spinach, soybean oil, grapes, and hard-boiled eggs. Vitamin K2 can be obtained from meat, as well as dairy products like cheese and eggs.

Ongoing Research on Vitamin K

& Its Effects on Diseases

Although people believe that Vitamin K can help in treating the following diseases, there is little evidence to support this assertion.

Breast Cancer Prevention

Some research suggests that Vitamin K2, in a higher dietary intake, may be linked with a reduced risk of developing breast cancer in women. However, further research is required before this can be said for certain.

Overall Cancer Prevention

Some research have stated that adequate intake of Vitamin K2 is directly linked with a reduced risk for death due to cancer. But it may not be linked to a prevention of any kind of cancer. Vitamin K1, on the other hand, does not seem to be linked with either cancer-related deaths or cancer prevention.

Prevention of Heart Diseases

There is some research to suggest that a adequate dose of Vitamin K2 can be associated with a lower risk of coronary calcification. It occurs in cases where a layer of plaque is developed in the inner lining of the coronary arteries. It is suggested that Vitamin K is also linked to a lower risk of death that is caused by coronary heart diseases. Still, there is evidence that suggests that taking Vitamin K1 from medication may reduce or prevent the advancement of coronary calcification.

Prevention of Cystic Fibrosis

People who are suffering from cystic fibrosis may have a low level of Vitamin K due to problems that are related to digesting fat. People who have trouble digesting fat, and are suffering from cystic fibrosis, may take a combination of Vitamins A, D, E and K, in order to improve the level of Vitamin K in their body.

Research also suggests that taking Vitamin K orally can enhance the production of osteocalcin, which plays a major role in building the bones in the body and in regulating the metabolism.

Prevention of Diabetes

There is enough research to suggest that taking multivitamins is a better option in lowering the risk of developing diabetes but not Vitamin K1.

Prevention of High Cholesterol

The benefits of Vitamin K2 in reducing high cholesterol is limited to a certain type of condition. Studies suggest that Vitamin K2 might lower the level of cholesterol in people who are on dialysis.

Prevention of Liver and Lung Cancer

Even after the curative treatment of cancer, it seems that Vitamin K2 does not prevent cancer from recurring. But some research shows that Vitamin K2 might help in the prevention of the development of liver cancer in people who are suffering from liver cirrhosis.

Some research suggest that a higher intake of Vitamin K2 is directly linked with a reduced risk of developing lung cancer and deaths related to lung cancer. However, intake of Vitamin K1 does not seem to prevent lung cancer or deaths related to lung cancer.

Health Benefits of Vitamin K

Improves Bone Health

Researchers have studied Vitamin K thoroughly and they have found that there is a correlation between low levels of Vitamin K and osteoporosis. Numerous studies and research have suggested that Vitamin K supports and maintains strong bones, improves bone density, and decreases the risks associated with fractures.

Improves Cognitive Health

Scientists have conducted studies that show that among older adults, increased blood levels of Vitamin K have been linked with improved episodic memory. The results of one study showed that individuals who are still healthy after the age of 70 years and who have adequate concentrations of Vitamin K1 in their systems showed the highest levels of verbal episodic memory.

Improves Heart Health

Vitamin K helps our body maintain regular blood pressure by preventing mineralization. Because of this, the heart can freely pump blood through the whole body. Mineralization is something that occurs naturally with age, and it is a major risk factor for diseases related to the heart in humans. Adequate levels of Vitamin K have been shown to reduce the risk of strokes.

Side Effects of Vitamin K

Vitamin K is safe for women who are pregnant or breastfeeding, as long as it is taken in the recommended quantities. It is recommended that a Vitamin K doses be taken only after consulting the doctor.

The form of Vitamin K known as Vitamin K1 is safe for children if taken orally, or by injection.

Taking more Vitamin K than necessary can lead to kidney-related diseases, especially if a person is receiving dialysis treatment.

People who take Vitamin K and have decreased bile

secretion should also take supplementary bile salts. These should be taken along with Vitamin K in order to make sure that it is absorbed completely by the body.

Symptoms of Vitamin K Deficiency

There are symptoms that point toward the deficiency of Vitamin K. These symptoms include, but are not limited to bruising, oozing from nose or gums, uncontrolled bleeding from wounds, injection or surgical sites, heavy menstrual periods, bleeding from the gastrointestinal tract, and bleeding present in urine or stool.

Dosage of Vitamin K

Although most people get enough Vitamin K from foods, the recommended daily consumption based on age is as follows:

- For children of up to 12 months, 2.5 mcg/day.
- For children between the age of 1 and 3, 30 mcg/day.
- For children from 4 to 8, 55 mcg/day.
- For age 9 to 13, 60 mcg/day.

- For girls 14 to 18, 75 mcg/day.
- For women 19 and older, 90 mcg/day.
- For boys 14 to 18, 75 mcg/day.
- For men 19 and above, 120 mcg/day.

These doses are not separate from the amounts that can be obtained from food sources. The intake of Vitamin K from food and other sources should not exceed these limits. It is dangerous to have an excess of Vitamin K in the body.

We have seen the advantages and the disadvantages of Vitamins K1 and K2. As has been suggested earlier, everything in adequate quantities is good, but anything more than that can cause problems, and even severe diseases. It is always best to consult a doctor before taking supplements or drugs containing Vitamin K. Vitamin K helps in many ways, but there is still research and studies that need to be conducted on this Vitamin.

After reading the whole book, I hope that you now know more about Vitamins and their benefits for the overall health of humans. Vitamins, although taken in small quantities, can perform miracles in our bodies. We have learned that Vitamins can be found in vegetables, fruits, nuts, oils, and even in animals, apart from other products like moisturizers.

There are numerous benefits of ingesting adequate amounts of Vitamins. Vitamins greatly improve eyesight and other systems in our bodies.

Vitamins play a major role in the respiratory system, bones, and in making the immune system stronger. They also help in improving the nervous system of our body, provide our body with the energy to do various tasks, and they also widen the blood vessels and prevent heart-related diseases.

Other benefits of Vitamins include improving liver functions, metabolism, circulatory system, and blood formation process. They participate directly in the formation of red blood cells and are an essential source for genetic material.

Vitamins also make our bones and teeth strong. They help regulate and improve the menstrual cycle, the neurological functions, and also keeps the skin moisturized.

From everything that we have read, it can be concluded that Vitamins are essential for our body, not just in maintaining good health, but also in improving our health. The deficiencies of Vitamins can lead to serious problems, so it is recommended that we give our body the Vitamins it needs in order to stay healthy. It is also notable that we should not take more than the required dosage of Vitamins to avoid problems resulting from Vitamins overdose.

Bibliography

Vitamin A in the treatment of Renal Disease (2018) Retrieved from https://academic.oup.com/ndt/article/16/10/2111/1866274

Thiamine deficiency and nervous system function disturbances (2018) Retrieved From https://www.ncbi.nlm.nih.gov/pubmed/4029224

Maternal periconceptional folic acid intake and risk of autism spectrum disorders and developmental delay in the CHARGE (CHildhood Autism Risks from Genetics and Environment) case-control study (30 May, 2012) Retrieved from https://academic.oup.com/ajcn/article/96/1/80/4571464

What is rheumatoid arthritis? (2004-2018) Retrieved from https://www.medicalnewstoday.com/articles/323361.php

Methotrexate: Managing Side Effects, Understand the side effects of methotrexate and how you can take measures to keep them to a minimum. (2018) Retrieved from https://www.arthritis.org/living-with-arthritis/treatments/medication/drug-types/disease-modifying-drugs/methotrexate-side-effects.php

Folic acid (2018) Retrieved from https://www.marchofdimes.org/pregnancy/folic-acid.aspx

The impact of mandatory fortification of flour with folic acid on the blood folate levels of an Australian population (17 January, 2011) Retrieved From https://www.mja.com.au/journal/2011/194/2/impact-mandatory-fortification-flour-folic-acid-blood-folate-levels-australian \

What to know about cancer (2004-2018) Retrieved from https://www.medicalnewstoday.com/articles/323648.php

What is depression and what can I do about it? (2004-2018) Retrieved from https://www.medicalnewstoday.com/kc/depression-causes-symptoms-treatments-8933

Relationships between folate and inflammatory features of asthma (March, 2013) Retrieved from https://www.ncbi.nlm.nih.gov/pmc/articles/PMC4016954/

Memory and Motor Coordination Improvement by Folic Acid Supplementation in Healthy Adult Male Rats (2018) Retrieved from https://www.ncbi.nlm.nih.gov/pmc/articles/PMC3646228/

Effect of folic acid on bone metabolism: a randomized double blind clinical trial in postmenopausal osteoporotic women (16 September, 2014) Retrieved from https://www.ncbi.nlm.nih.gov/pmc/articles/PMC4172791/

Folate Deficiency (13 November, 2018) Retrieved from https://medlineplus.gov/ency/article/000354.htm

Listing of Vitamins (14 august, 2017) Retrieved from https://www.health.harvard.edu/newsweek/Listing_of_Vitamins.htm

Vitamins: what are they and what they do? (26 September, 2017) Retrieved from https://www.medicalnewstoday.com/articles/195878.php

Collagen: what are they and what are they uses? (16 June, 2017) Retrieved from https://www.medicalnewstoday.com/articles/262881.php

How can antioxidants benefit our health? (29 May, 2018) Retrieved form https://www.medicalnewstoday.com/articles/301506.php

Everything you need to know about scurvy (6 December, 2017) Retrieved from https://www.medicalnewstoday.com/articles/155758.php

Everything you need to know about anemia (28 November, 2017) Retrieved from https://www.medicalnewstoday.com/articles/158800.php

Fatigue: why am I so tired and what can I do about it? (16 August, 2017) Retrieved from https://www.medicalnewstoday.com/articles/248002.php

Vitamin and human wound healing. (2018) Retrieved from https://www.ncbi.nlm.nih.gov/pubmed/7038579

Everything you need to know about inflammation (24 November, 2017) Retrieved from https://www.medicalnewstoday.com/articles/248423.php

All you need to know about tuberculosis (27 November, 2017) Retrieved from https://www.medicalnewstoday.com/articles/8856.php

Mycobacterium tuberculosis is extraordinarily sensitive to killing by a Vitamin C-included Fenton reaction (2018) Retrieved from https://www.ncbi.nlm.nih.gov/pmc/articles/PMC3698613/

What to know about radiation therapy? (16 February, 2018) Retrieved from https://www.medicalnewstoday.com/articles/158513.php

Everything you need to know about heart disease (7

February, 2018) Retrieved from https://www.medicalnewstoday.com/articles/237191.php

Everything you need to know about hypertension (11 December, 2017) Retrieved from https://www.medicalnewstoday.com/articles/150109.php

What's to know about high blood pressure (28 November, 2017) Retrieved from https://www.medicalnewstoday.com/articles/159283.php

What causes high cholesterol? (27 November, 2017) Retrieved from https://www.medicalnewstoday.com/articles/9152.php

What you need to know about cataracts (19 December, 2017) Retrieved from https://www.medicalnewstoday.com/articles/157510.php

What is age-related macular degeneration (AMD)? (7 June 2018) Retrieved from https://www.medicalnewstoday.com/articles/15210

5.php

Antihistamine effect of supplemental ascorbic acid and neutrophil chemotaxis (2018) Retrieved from https://www.ncbi.nlm.nih.gov/pubmed/1578094

Placebos: The power of the placebo effect (7 September, 2017) Retrieved from https://www.medicalnewstoday.com/articles/306437.php

Vitamin C selectively kills *KRAS* and *BRAF* mutant colorectal cancer cells by targeting GAPDH (2018) Retrieved from http://science.sciencemag.org/content/350/6266/1391

High dose Vitamin C and Cancer: Has Linus pauling been vindicated? (18 August, 2018) Retrieved from https://sciencebasedmedicine.org/high-dose-Vitamin-c-and-cancer-has-linus-pauling-been-vindicated/

Dr. Ronald Hoffman, Intravenous Vitamin C for cancer (2018) Retrieved from http://www.hoffmancenter.com/page.cfm/783?Template=Default_Print

Antihistamine effect of supplemental ascorbic acid and neutrophil chemotaxis (2018) Retrieved from https://www.ncbi.nlm.nih.gov/pubmed/1578094

Identification of Vitamin C transporters in the human airways: a cross-sectional in vivo study (2018) Retrieved from https://bmjopen.bmj.com/content/5/4/e006979.short

Vitamin C, Vitamin and minerals (2018) Retrieved from https://www.nhs.uk/conditions/Vitamins-and-minerals/Vitamin-c/

What you should know about diarrhea (28 November, 2017) Retrieved from https://www.medicalnewstoday.com/articles/158634.php

How do you get kidney stones? (29 November, 2017) Retrieved from https://www.medicalnewstoday.com/articles/154193.php

Everything you need to know about menopause (28 September, 2017) Retrieved from https://www.medicalnewstoday.com/articles/155651.php

Iron overload disorder: All you need to know (9 March, 2017) Retrieved from https://www.medicalnewstoday.com/articles/166455.php

Osteoporosis explained (4 January, 2018) Retrieved from https://www.medicalnewstoday.com/articles/155646.php

Calcium: Health benefits, foods, and Deficiency (21 August, 2017) Retrieved from https://www.medicalnewstoday.com/articles/248958.php

Everything you need to know about Rickets (19 December, 2017) Retrieved from https://www.medicalnewstoday.com/articles/176941.php

All you need to know about flu (20 December, 2017) Retrieved from https://www.medicalnewstoday.com/articles/176941.php

Vitamin D's Role in Health — Deterministic or Indeterminate? By Stephanie Dunne and Jenna A. Bell, PhD, RD Today's

Dietitian (2018) Retrieved from https://www.todaysdietitian.com/newarchives/070114p48.shtml

Type 2 Diabetes: causes and symptoms (2016) Retrieved from https://www.medicalnewstoday.com/info/diabetes/type2diabetes.php

What is normal blood pressure (2017) Retrieved from https://www.medicalnewstoday.com/articles/270644.php

A 16-week randomized clinical trial of 2000 international units daily Vitamin D3 supplementation in black youth: 25-hydroxyVitamin D, adiposity, and arterial stiffness. (2018) Retrieved from https://www.ncbi.nlm.nih.gov/pubmed/20660028

Vitamin D in Atopic Dermatitis, Asthma and Allergic Diseases (2018) Retrieved from https://www.ncbi.nlm.nih.gov/pmc/articles/PMC2914320/

What is asthma? (2018) Retrieved from https://www.medicalnewstoday.com/articles/323523.php

What to know about eczema? (2017) Retrieved from https://www.medicalnewstoday.com/articles/14417.php

Everything you need to know about preeclampsia (2017) Retrieved from https://www.medicalnewstoday.com/articles/252025.php

What is cesarean delivery? (2018) Retrieved from https://www.medicalnewstoday.com/articles/299502.php

Bacterial vaginosis: Causes, symptoms, and treatments. (2018) Retrieved from https://www.medicalnewstoday.com/articles/184622.php

Alopecia areata: Causes, symptoms, and treatment. (2018) Retrieved from https://www.medicalnewstoday.com/articles/70956.php

Alzheimer's disease: Symptoms, stages, causes, and treatment. (2018) Retrieved, from https://www.medicalnewstoday.com/articles/159442.php

Am I Obese? How Experts Define What Obesity Is. (2018) retrieved from https://www.webmd.com/diet/obesity/features/am-i-obese#1

Bacterial vaginosis: Causes, symptoms, and treatments. (2018) Retrieved from https://www.medicalnewstoday.com/articles/184622.php

Celiac Disease. (2018) Retrieved from https://www.webmd.com/digestive-disorders/celiac-disease/default.htm

Chronic fatigue syndrome: Symptoms, treatment, and causes. (2018) Retrieved from https://www.medicalnewstoday.com/articles/184802.php

Colon cancer: Symptoms, treatment, and causes. (2018) Retrieved from https://www.medicalnewstoday.com/articles/150496.php

Crohns Disease. (2018) Retrieved from https://www.webmd.com/ibd-crohns-disease/crohns-disease/default.htm

Fatigue: Why am I so tired and what can I do about it? (2018) Retrieved from https://www.medicalnewstoday.com/articles/248002.php

Fibromyalgia: Symptoms, causes, and treatment. (2018) Retrieved from https://www.medicalnewstoday.com/articles/147083.php

Hoffman, M., & MD. The Kidneys: Picture, Function, Conditions, Tests, Treatments. (2018) Retrieved from https://www.webmd.com/kidney-stones/picture-of-the-kidneys

How much should I weigh for my height and age? BMI calculator and chart, waist-hip ratio. (2018) Retrieved from https://www.medicalnewstoday.com/articles/323446.php

Naeem, Z. Vitamin D Deficiency- An Ignored Epidemic. *International Journal of Health Sciences*, (2010). Retrieved from https://www.ncbi.nlm.nih.gov/pmc/articles/PMC3068797/

Quiz: How Well Do You Know Your Kidneys? (2018) Retrieved from https://www.webmd.com/a-to-z-guides/rm-quiz-kidneys

Quiz: How Well Do You Know Your Liver? (2018) Retrieved from https://www.webmd.com/hepatitis/rmq-know-your-liver

Rheumatoid arthritis (RA): Symptoms, causes, and complications. (2018) Retrieved from https://www.medicalnewstoday.com/articles/323361.php

Slideshow: What Can I Eat? A Guide for New Vegetarians. (2018) Retrieved from https://www.webmd.com/diet/ss/slideshow-vegetarian-diet

Swine flu: Causes, symptoms, and treatment. (2018) Retrieved from https://www.medicalnewstoday.com/articles/147720.php

Vitamin D 101 — A Detailed Beginner's Guide. (11 January, 2015). Retrieved from https://www.healthline.com/nutrition/Vitamin-d-

Vitamin D and Cancer — Evidence Suggests This Vital Nutrient May Cut Risk. (2018) Retrieved, from https://www.todaysdietitian.com/newarchives/1001 12p58.shtml

Weisse, K., Winkler, S., Hirche, F., Herberth, G., Hinz, D., Bauer, M., ... Lehmann, I. Maternal and newborn Vitamin D status and its impact on food allergy development in the German LINA cohort study (2013) Retrieved from https://doi.org/10.1111/all.12081

What Is Cystic Fibrosis? What Causes It? (2018) Retrieved, from https://www.webmd.com/children/what-is-cystic-fibrosis

www.ingramcontent.com/pod-product-compliance
Lightning Source LLC
Chambersburg PA
CBHW021401210526
45463CB00001B/189